T0226959

Infection in the Intensive Care Unit

Editors

TODD M. TARTAVOULLE
JENNIFER MANNING

CRITICAL CARE NURSING CLINICS OF NORTH AMERICA

www.ccnursing.theclinics.com

Consulting Editor
JAN FOSTER

March 2017 • Volume 29 • Number 1

ELSEVIER

1600 John F. Kennedy Boulevard • Suite 1800 • Philadelphia, Pennsylvania, 19103-2899

http://www.theclinics.com

CRITICAL CARE NURSING CLINICS OF NORTH AMERICA Volume 29, Number 1
March 2017 ISSN 0899-5885, ISBN-13: 978-0-323-47737-6

Editor: Kerry Holland
Developmental Editor: Colleen Dietzler

© 2017 Elsevier Inc. All rights reserved.

This periodical and the individual contributions contained in it are protected under copyright by Elsevier, and the following terms and conditions apply to their use:

Photocopying
Single photocopies of single articles may be made for personal use as allowed by national copyright laws. Permission of the Publisher and payment of a fee is required for all other photocopying, including multiple or systematic copying, copying for advertising or promotional purposes, resale, and all forms of document delivery. Special rates are available for educational institutions that wish to make photocopies for non-profit educational classroom use. For information on how to seek permission visit www.elsevier.com/permissions or call: (+44) 1865 843830 (UK)/(+1) 215 239 3804 (USA).

Derivative Works
Subscribers may reproduce tables of contents or prepare lists of articles including abstracts for internal circulation within their institutions. Permission of the Publisher is required for resale or distribution outside the institution. Permission of the Publisher is required for all other derivative works, including compilations and translations (please consult www.elsevier.com/permissions).

Electronic Storage or Usage
Permission of the Publisher is required to store or use electronically any material contained in this periodical, including any article or part of an article (please consult www.elsevier.com/permissions). Except as outlined above, no part of this publication may be reproduced, stored in a retrieval system or transmitted in any form or by any means, electronic, mechanical, photocopying, recording or otherwise, without prior written permission of the Publisher.

Notice
No responsibility is assumed by the Publisher for any injury and/or damage to persons or property as a matter of products liability, negligence or otherwise, or from any use or operation of any methods, products, instructions or ideas contained in the material herein. Because of rapid advances in the medical sciences, in particular, independent verification of diagnoses and drug dosages should be made.

Although all advertising material is expected to conform to ethical (medical) standards, inclusion in this publication does not constitute a guarantee or endorsement of the quality or value of such product or of the claims made of it by its manufacturer.

Critical Care Nursing Clinics of North America (ISSN 0899-5885) is published quarterly by Elsevier Inc., 360 Park Avenue South, New York, NY 10010-1710. Months of issue are March, June, September, and December. Business and Editorial Offices: 1600 John F. Kennedy Blvd., Suite 1800, Philadelphia, PA 19103-2899. Periodicals postage paid at New York, NY and additional mailing offices. Subscription prices are $155.00 per year for US individuals, $385.00 per year for US institutions, $100.00 per year for US students and residents, $200.00 per year for Canadian individuals, $483.00 per year for Canadian institutions, $230.00 per year for international individuals, $483.00 per year for international institutions and $115.00 per year for Canadian and international students/residents. To receive student/resident rate, orders must be accompanied by name of affiliated institution, data of term, and the *signature* of program/residency coordinator on institution letterhead. Orders will be billed at individual rate until proof of status is received. Foreign air speed delivery is included in all *Clinics* subscription prices. All prices are subject to change without notice. **POSTMASTER:** Send address changes to *Critical Care Nursing Clinics of North America*, Elsevier Health Sciences Division, Subscription Customer Service, 3251 Riverport Lane, Maryland Heights, MO 63043. **Customer Service: 1-800-654-2452 (US and Canada); 314-447-8871 (outside US and Canada). Fax: 314-447-8029. E-mail:** JournalsCustomerService-usa@elsevier.com **(for print support) and** JournalsOnlineSupport-usa@elsevier.com **(for online support).**

Reprints. For copies of 100 or more of articles in this publication, please contact the Commercial Reprints Department, Elsevier Inc., 360 Park Avenue South, New York, New York, 10010-1710; Tel.: 212-633-3874, Fax: 212-633-3820, and E-mail: reprints@elsevier.com.

Critical Care Nursing Clinics of North America is covered in *MEDLINE/PubMed (Index Medicus), International Nursing Index, Nursing Citation Index, Cumulative Index to Nursing and Allied Health Literature, and RNdex Top 100.*

Contributors

CONSULTING EDITOR

JAN FOSTER, PhD, APRN, CNS
Formerly, Associate Professor, College of Nursing, Texas Woman's University, Houston; President, Nursing Inquiry and Intervention, Inc, The Woodlands, Texas

EDITORS

TODD M. TARTAVOULLE, DNS, APRN, CNS-BC
Assistant Professor of Clinical Nursing, School of Nursing, Louisiana State University Health Sciences Center, New Orleans, Louisiana

JENNIFER MANNING, DNS, APRN, CNS, CNE
Associate Dean for Undergraduate Nursing Programs, Nursing Department, School of Nursing, Louisiana State University Health Sciences Center, Louisiana Center for Promotion of Optimal Health Outcomes: A JBI Center of Excellence, New Orleans, Louisiana

AUTHORS

JENNIFER E. BADEAUX, DNP, CRNA, APRN
Assistant Professor, Nurse Anesthesia Program, School of Nursing, Louisiana State University Health Sciences Center, New Orleans, Louisiana

KENDRA M. BARRIER, PhD, RN, MSN
Assistant Dean of Student Services, Instructor, School of Nursing, Louisiana State University Health Sciences Center, New Orleans, Louisiana

CHRISTINE BOEV, PhD, RN, CCRN, CNE
Assistant Professor of Nursing, St. John Fisher College Wegmans School of Nursing, Nurse, Pediatric Cardiac Care Center, Golisano Children's Hospital, Strong Memorial Hospital, University of Rochester, Rochester, New York

JEAN E. CEFALU, PhD, APRN, AGNP-C, CWOCN, CFCN, CNE
Adult-Gerontology Primary Care Nurse Practitioner Program Coordinator, Instructor, Nursing Department, School of Nursing, Louisiana State University Health Sciences Center, New Orleans, Louisiana

ALISON H. DAVIS, PhD, RN, CHSE
Director of Nursing Skills and Technology Center, Assistant Professor, School of Nursing, Louisiana State University Health Sciences Center, New Orleans, Louisiana

LATANJA DIVENS, DNP, APRN, FNP-BC
Nurse Practitioner Nephrology Course Coordinator, School of Nursing, Louisiana State University Health Sciences Center, New Orleans, Louisiana

LEANNE H. FOWLER, DNP, MBA, AGACNP-BC, CCRN, CNE
BSN to DNP Adult/Gerontology Acute Care Nurse Practitioner Program Director, School of Nursing, Louisiana State University Health Sciences Center, New Orleans, Louisiana

DEBORAH D. GARBEE, PhD, APRN, ACNS-BC
Associate Dean Professional Practice, Community Service, and Advanced Practice Nursing, Department of Adult Health Nursing, School of Nursing, Louisiana State University Health Sciences Center, Louisiana Center for Promotion of Optimal Health Outcomes: A JBI Center of Excellence, New Orleans, Louisiana

MISTY JENKINS, MSN, APRN, ACNP-BC, CCRN
Acute Care Nurse Practitioner, Pulmonary Critical Care, Ochsner Medical Center, New Orleans, Louisiana

NICOLE J. JONES, MN, RN-BC, APRN, ACNS-BC, CCNS, CHFN
Clinical Nurse Specialist, Cardiology Care Performance Improvement Department, East Jefferson General Hospital, Metairie, Louisiana

ELIZABETH KISS, DNP, FNP-BC, RN
Assistant Professor of Nursing, St. John Fisher College Wegmans School of Nursing, Nurse Practitioner, Surgical Cancer Center, Wilmot Cancer Center, Strong Memorial Hospital, University of Rochester, Rochester, New York

SUSAN LEE, MSN, APRN, FNP-BC
Critical Care Simulation Course Coordinator, School of Nursing, Louisiana State University Health Sciences Center, New Orleans, Louisiana

JENNIFER MANNING, DNS, APRN, CNS, CNE
Associate Dean for Undergraduate Nursing Programs, Nursing Department, School of Nursing, Louisiana State University Health Sciences Center, Louisiana Center for Promotion of Optimal Health Outcomes: A JBI Center of Excellence, New Orleans, Louisiana

JENNIFER B. MARTIN, DNP, CRNA, APRN
Instructor, Nurse Anesthesia Program, School of Nursing, Louisiana State University Health Sciences Center, New Orleans, Louisiana

STEPHANIE S. PIERCE, PhD, RN, CNE
Program Director of Nurse Educator Program, Program Director of Career Alternative RN Education and Program Director of Articulation Programs, Department of Community Health Nursing, School of Nursing, Louisiana State University Health Sciences Center, Louisiana Center for Promotion of Optimal Health Outcomes: A JBI Center of Excellence, New Orleans, Louisiana

TODD M. TARTAVOULLE, DNS, APRN, CNS-BC
Assistant Professor of Clinical Nursing, School of Nursing, Louisiana State University Health Sciences Center, New Orleans, Louisiana

CHLOE D. VILLAVASO, MN, RN, APRN, ACNS-BC
Clinical Nurse Specialist, Cardiology Care Performance Improvement Department, East Jefferson General Hospital, Metairie, Louisiana

FIONA WINTERBOTTOM, DNP, MSN, APRN, ACNS-BC, CCRN
Clinical Nurse Specialist, Pulmonary Critical Care, Ochsner Medical Center, New Orleans, Louisiana

Contents

> The incidence of surgical site infections (SSIs) has a significant negative impact on health care. SSIs are associated with increased mortality, cost, readmissions, and prolonged length of stay. Although recent data show a 17% decrease in the incidence of SSIs among acute care hospitals in the United States, mortality related to SSIs remains clinically significant. The interprofessional team is a critical structure in evaluating surgical practices and outcomes and new evidence-based practices to direct education, interventions, and communication of SSI prevention strategies.

> Pulmonary arterial hypertension is a lethal condition, and the management of sepsis in patients with pulmonary arterial hypertension is challenging. As the disease progresses, the right ventricle is susceptible to failure due to a high pulmonary vascular resistance. The limited ability of the right ventricle to increase cardiac output in septic shock makes it difficult to deliver oxygen to the organ and tissues. Intravascular volume replacement and vasoactive drugs should only be considered after a thorough assessment. Priorities of care include improving cardiac output and oxygen delivery by optimizing preload, reducing afterload, and improving contractility.

> Many challenges exist in caring for older adults with infection in critical care environments. Older adults are at high risk due to diminished reserve, age-related changes, comorbidities, subtle clinical presentations, and institutionalization. Additional risks include infections, such as pneumonia, influenza, and nosocomial infections. Age-related changes contribute to the increased risk of infection in older adults. Nursing assessments should be tailored to the needs of the older patient. To improve health care outcomes in this population, nursing care of the critically ill older adult with infection should include comprehensive assessment, surveillance for risks, and strategies aimed to aggressively treat infection.

The patient with sepsis in the setting of hepatitis C virus (HCV)-related
cirrhosis can have a more rapid decline in other organ dysfunction during
critical illness and faces further increase in the risk for death. This article
discusses the role of liver function in the patient with a systemic critical
illness in contrast to the worsened pathophysiology of the patient with
cirrhosis secondary to chronic HCV infection and critical illness, inpatient
and posthospitalization management of the critically ill patient with chronic
HCV-related cirrhosis, and the nursing implications and recommendations
for future research for this population.

Health care–associated infections (HAIs) are the primary cause of preventable death and disability among hospitalized patients. According to the
Centers for Disease Control and Prevention (CDC), complications or infections secondary to either device implantation or surgery are referred to as
HAIs. Specifically, the CDC monitors surgical site infections, central-line–
associated bloodstream infection, catheter-associated urinary tract infections, and ventilator-associated pneumonias. This article explores HAIs
specific to pathophysiology, epidemiology, and prevention, and how
nurses can work together with other health care providers to decrease
the incidence of these preventable complications.

Fungal infections are rare compared with bacterial infections, but they are
on the increase in critical care units. Diagnosis can be difficult, resulting in
increased mortality. Immunocompromised patients are at higher risk for
fungal infections, including organ transplant, oncology, and HIV/AIDS patients. Fatigue and fever are common symptoms that require critical care
nurses to remain vigilant in assessment to identify at-risk patients and promote use of timely cultures and appropriate treatments for fungal infections. Critical care nurses can contribute to decreasing risk for fungal
infections by controlling glucose levels, decreasing the use of invasive
lines, and preventing unnecessary antibiotic use.

Patients admitted to critical care units are at high risk for increased
morbidity and mortality from skin and deep wound infections. Despite
considerable progress, wound healing remains a challenge to many clinicians. Nurses working in critical care environments need to understand the
anatomic and physiologic basis for wound healing, distinguish wound
inflammation from wound infection, recognize the presence of biofilms,
and implement evidence-based wound care in order to promote successful outcomes in this patient population.

Solid organ transplantation has become a well-established standard of care for end-organ failure, and the nurse in the intensive care unit may be exposed to these patients at any stage in the care continuum of pretransplant or posttransplant care. Knowledge of risk factors, timing, and treatments for infections may help to enhance clinical practices and optimize patient safety and clinical outcomes.

Isolates from ICUs most commonly find multidrug-resistant (MDR) gram-negative bacteria. The purpose of this article is to discuss the significant impact MDR gram-negative infections are having on ICUs, the threat on health and mortality, and effective and new approaches aimed to combat MDR gram-negative infections in critically ill populations. Inappropriate antibiotic therapies for suspected or documented infections are the leading cause of the emergence of bacterial resistance. A variety of strategies are aimed at combatting this international burden via antibiotic stewardship programs. Studies are demonstrating promise against the virulence MDR gram-negative infections have posed.

Sepsis and severe sepsis are leading causes of death in the United States and the most common causes of death among critically ill patients in noncoronary intensive care units. Diagnosis of infection and sepsis is a subjective clinical judgment based on the criteria for systemic inflammatory reaction, which is highly sensitive, not specific, and often misleading in intensively treated patients. Biomarkers are emerging as adjuncts to traditional diagnostic measures. No biomarkers have sufficient specificity or sensitivity to be routinely used in clinical practice, but they can aid in the diagnosis and treatment of infection versus inflammation.

CRITICAL CARE NURSING
CLINICS OF NORTH AMERICA

THE CLINICS ARE AVAILABLE ONLINE!
Access your subscription at:
www.theclinics.com

Preface

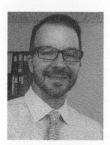 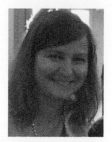

Todd M. Tartavoulle, DNS, APRN, CNS-BC   Jennifer Manning, DNS, APRN, CNS, CNE
Editors

Intensive care units account for fewer than 10% of total beds in most hospitals. More than 20% of all nosocomial infections are acquired in intensive care units. Hospitals have implemented quality improvement initiatives to decrease infection; however, incidence of nosocomial infections has increased, causing an increase in hospital care cost of a patient by $10,375 and an increase in length of stay by 3.3 days. An estimated annual cost of 9.8 billion dollars has been spent treating nosocomial infections.

Patients in an intensive care unit have a greater risk of acquiring a nosocomial infection than those in non-critical care areas. The predominant types of infection and the ecology of potential pathogens vary between different intensive care units. The variance in different pathogens among intensive care units may be attributed to patient and case mix, device utilization rates, teaching affiliations, and empirical antibiotic usage patterns. Trauma patients, chronic illness patients, and transplant patients have unique predispositions to different infections.

Todd M. Tartavoulle, DNS, APRN, CNS-BC
School of Nursing
Louisiana State University Health Sciences Center
1900 Gravier Street
New Orleans, LA 70112, USA

Jennifer Manning, DNS, APRN, CNS, CNE
Nursing Department
School of Nursing
Louisiana State University Health Sciences Center
1900 Gravier Street
Office 4B17
New Orleans, LA 70112, USA

E-mail addresses:
ttarta@lsuhsc.edu (T.M. Tartavoulle)
jmanni@lsuhsc.edu (J. Manning)

Crit Care Nurs Clin N Am 29 (2017) ix
http://dx.doi.org/10.1016/j.cnc.2016.12.001
0899-5885/17/© 2016 Published by Elsevier Inc.

An Interprofessional Team Approach to Decreasing Surgical Site Infection After Coronary Artery Bypass Graft Surgery

Nicole J. Jones, MN, RN-BC, APRN, ACNS-BC, CCNS, CHFN*,
Chloe D. Villavaso, MN, RN, APRN, ACNS-BC

KEYWORDS

- Coronary artery bypass • Surgical wound infection (prevention and control)
- Surgical site infection prevention strategies

KEY POINTS

- Surgical site infection (SSI) after coronary artery bypass graft (CABG) surgery has profound effects on patient outcomes, including mortality, cost, readmissions, and length of stay.
- Approximately 60% of SSIs are preventable through use of evidence-based strategies.
- A highly collaborative interprofessional team facilitates evaluation and implementation of recommended and novel strategies.
- Many strategies can be hardwired for clinicians to prevent SSI.

INCIDENCE OF SURGICAL SITE INFECTION AND IMPACT ON OUTCOMES

The incidence of SSIs has a significant negative impact on health care. SSIs are associated with increased mortality, cost, readmissions, and prolonged length of stay.[1] SSIs account for 31% of all hospital-acquired infections, making them one of the most costly and most common hospital-acquired infections.[2,3] The incidence of SSIs in the United States is approximately 160,000 to 300,000 annually, and SSIs occur in 2% to 5% of inpatient surgeries.[3] Although recent data show a 17% decrease in the incidence of SSIs among acute care hospitals in the United States, mortality related to SSIs remains clinically significant.[4] SSIs have a mortality rate of 3%.[2] Patients who develop an SSI have up to an 11 times higher risk of death compared with surgical

Disclosure Statement: The authors have nothing to disclose.
Cardiology Care Performance Improvement Department, East Jefferson General Hospital, 4200 Houma Boulevard, Metairie, LA 70006, USA
* Corresponding author.
E-mail address: njjones@ejgh.org

Crit Care Nurs Clin N Am 29 (2017) 1–13
http://dx.doi.org/10.1016/j.cnc.2016.09.001
0899-5885/17/© 2016 Elsevier Inc. All rights reserved.

patients who do not develop an SSI.[3] Of the 700,000 cardiac surgeries performed in the United States each year, more than 67% are CABG surgeries.[5] Mediastinitis occurs in 5% of all cardiac surgeries and is associated with a 40% risk of mortality.[5]

SSIs add an estimated $38,000 to the cost of an admission,[6] which adds $3 billion to $10 billion in US health care costs each year.[3] This increase in cost is related to the additional care required to treat these infections, including prolonged acute care and critical care hospital stays.[7] Seven to eleven additional hospital days have been associated with every SSI.[7] Hospital readmissions related to SSIs can have a significant financial impact on health care organizations. The rate of SSI readmission is between 11% and 16.5%[8,9] and costs 3 times as much as readmissions unrelated to major infections.[6] Due to the significant impact SSIs have on the outcomes of patients, the US Centers for Disease Control and Prevention (CDC) National Healthcare Safety Network has established the goal of 30% reduction in SSI admission and readmission by 2020.[10]

DEFINITION OF SURGICAL SITE INFECTION

The CDC provides extensive instructions to infection preventionists to aid in the reporting of SSIs. These infections are classified according to the degree of tissue involvement and can range from superficial to organ/space involvement. The CDC's full SSI classification criteria can be accessed at http://www.cdc.gov/nhsn/PDFs/pscManual/9pscSSIcurrent.pdf.

An overview of the criteria to classify an SSI are as follows[2]:

1. Superficial incisional SSI—infection occurs within 30 days after the operative procedure and involves only the skin and subcutaneous tissue of the incision and at least 1 of the following:
   a. Purulent drainage from the superficial incision
   b. Organisms identified from an aseptically obtained specimen from the superficial incision or subcutaneous tissue
   c. Superficial incision that is deliberately opened by a physician, organism identified by culture, and at least 1 of the following signs or symptoms: pain or tenderness, localized swelling, erythema, or heat, unless the culture is negative
   d. Diagnosis of a superficial incisional SSI by the surgeon, attending physician, or designee
2. Deep incisional SSI—infection occurs within 90 days after the operative procedure and involves the deep soft tissues of the incision and at least one of the following:
   a. Purulent drainage from the deep incision
   b. A deep incision spontaneously dehisces or is deliberately opened or aspirated by a physician or designee and identified by culture and the patient has at least 1 of the following signs or symptoms: fever (>100.4°F), localized pain, or tenderness, unless the culture is negative
   c. An abscess or other evidence of infection involving the deep incision that is detected on gross anatomic or histopathologic examination or imaging test
3. Organ/space SSI—infection occurs within 90 days after the operative procedure and involves any part of the body deeper than the fascial/muscle layers that is opened or manipulated during the operative procedure and at least 1 of the following:
   a. Purulent drainage from a drain that is placed into the organ/space
   b. Organisms are identified from an aseptically obtained fluid or tissue in the organ/space by culture
   c. An abscess or other evidence of infection involving the organ/space that is detected on gross anatomic or histopathologic examination or imaging test

In addition to meeting these criteria for organ/space SSI, a postoperative CABG surgery patient must also meet at least 1 criterion for mediastinitis:

1. Organisms identified from mediastinal tissue or fluid by a culture or non–culture-based microbiologic testing method, which is performed for purposes of clinical diagnosis or treatment
2. Evidence of mediastinitis on gross anatomic or histopathologic examination
3. At least 1 of the following signs or symptoms: fever (>100.4°F), chest pain, or sternal instability (with no other recognizable cause) and at least 1 of the following
   a. Purulent drainage from mediastinal area
   b. Mediastinal widening on imaging test

RISK FACTORS FOR SURGICAL SITE INFECTION IN PATIENTS UNDERGOING CORONARY ARTERY BYPASS GRAFT

Numerous risk factors for developing SSIs after CABG have been identified. Advanced age and female gender are nonmodifiable risk factors for developing SSIs.[11,12] Comorbid conditions, such as obesity, diabetes, respiratory failure, heart failure, unstable angina, immunosuppression, chronic obstructive pulmonary disease, and renal impairment, increase the risk of SSIs.[11–14] Prolonged preoperative hospitalization, administration of inotropic agents, steroid use, hemodynamic support via intra-aortic balloon pump or ventricular assist device, and cardiogenic shock also pose a risk for developing SSIs.[11,12] Risk factors directly related to cardiac surgery include increased cardiopulmonary bypass time, length and complexity of surgery, bilateral internal mammary artery grafts, blood transfusions, synthetic aortic graft use, emergent or urgent surgery, and use of open saphenous vein harvest techniques.[11,12] Other risk factors identified in the literature include smoking, prolonged mechanical ventilation, postoperative sepsis, and the length of time between the onset of symptoms of infection and postoperative wound debridement.[11,12,14]

EVIDENCE-BASED SURGICAL SITE INFECTION PREVENTION STRATEGIES

According to Anderson and colleagues,[3] approximately 60% of SSIs can be prevented by implementing strategies included in evidence-based practice guidelines. The following sections of this article describe an interprofessional team approach to decreasing SSI after CABG, including current guidelines, SSI prevention strategies, and roles of interprofessional team members in preventing SSIs (**Box 1**).

Box 1
Evidence-based surgical site infection prevention strategies

- Appropriate hair removal
- Preoperative skin and nasal decolonization
- Meticulous hand hygiene
- Tissue optimization and skin preparation in the operating room
- Appropriate selection, dosage, timing, and duration of prophylactic antibiotics
- Maintenance of BG levels less than 180 mg/dL
- Surgical techniques
- Incisions covered with sterile dressing for 24 to 48 hours after surgery

---

Hair Removal

It has been widely accepted that hair removal should be avoided if possible before surgery. Use of razors creates tiny cuts in the skin, which promote further contamination of the skin with microorganisms and increase the risk of SSI.[3,15] If hair removal is necessary, clippers should be used on the morning of surgery.[15] As an alternative to clippers, depilatories may be used. Caution should be used with depilatories, due to the possibility of skin sensitivity reactions.[3,15]

Preoperative Skin Decolonization

Preoperative skin cleansing with chlorhexidine gluconate (CHG) has been proven to decrease the amount of bacteria on the skin but has not been definitively proven to decrease SSI in patients undergoing CABG.[3,16] Most guidelines list this intervention as reasonable. The 2014 update to the "Strategies to Prevent Surgical Site Infections in Acute Care Hospitals"[3] lists preoperative skin decolonization with CHG as an unresolved issue due to lack of evidence but states CHG-impregnated cloths have shown promise. Although the evidence linking the decolonization of the skin flora to decreased SSI may be questionable, some hospitals have used these CHG-impregnated cloths as a final skin cleansing to combat any nonadherence to preoperative bathing instructions and environmental microorganisms.

Hand Hygiene

The 2008 Association for Professionals in Infection Control and Epidemiology *Guide for the Prevention of Mediastinitis Surgical Site Infection Following Cardiac Surgery*[5] stresses the importance of hand hygiene for the intraoperative team and all caregivers. It includes case reports of 2 different infection outbreaks in this patient population, where 1 was linked to an anesthesiologist and the other was linked to ICU staff. Both outbreaks were resolved when the hand hygiene lapses were brought to the attention of the clinicians, and strict hand hygiene practices were implemented and enforced.[5] These reports underscore the importance of hand hygiene as one of the most simple yet effective SSI prevention strategies. Detailed information about hand hygiene and strategies to enhance adherence to strict and effective hand hygiene practices are included in the CDC "Guideline for Hand Hygiene in Health-Care Settings."[17] Additional information included in the guideline may serve as a hand hygiene gap analysis tool for intraoperative teams and all clinicians caring for CABG patients.

Tissue Optimization and Skin Preparation in the Operating Room

Tissue at the surgical site should be optimized by minimizing hypothermia and rewarming as early as possible. Administering supplemental oxygen decreases SSI by increasing the availability of oxygen at the tissue where the surgical incision will be made.[3] Skin should be prepared with an alcohol-containing decontaminant, and care should be taken to avoid pooling of the alcohol solution to prevent additional fire risk in the operating room. It is acceptable to use CHG-alcohol and povidone-iodine–alcohol preparations as skin disinfectants, because neither has proved superior in multiple studies.[3] These disinfectants have different instructions for application to the skin to maximize their effect on microorganisms during surgery. Surgery staff require ongoing education and surveillance with feedback to ensure optimal decontamination of the surgical site.

Antibiotic Prophylaxis

Guidelines published by the American Society of Health-System Pharmacists in 2013 recommend cefazolin or cefuroxime as first-line prophylactic antibiotic agents for

CABG.[18] If the duration of surgery exceeds 2 half-lives of the drug administered, a second dose is recommended.[18] Weight-based dosing of prophylactic antibiotics is also supported. Cefazolin (2 g) is recommended for patients weighing greater than 80 kg, and cefazolin (3 g) is recommended for patients weighing greater than 120 kg.[18] Some hospitals have standardized cefazolin for all adult patients at the 2 g dose. For patients who have a β-lactam allergy, vancomycin or clindamycin is recommended.[18] Vancomycin is also recommended for patients with known colonization with methicillin-resistant *Staphylococcus aureus* (MRSA).[18] If vancomycin is used as the prophylactic agent, the recommended dose is 15 mg/kg administered over 1 to 2 hours and given within 60 to 120 minutes of skin incision.[18] Vancomycin is not recommended for redosing during surgery, due to its longer half-life.[18] Caution is urged when using vancomycin as the sole prophylactic agent due to its narrower antimicrobial effectiveness.[18] When there is organizational evidence of SSIs caused by gram-negative organisms, clindamycin or vancomycin can be combined with cefazolin, aztreonam, aminoglycoside, or a single-dose fluoroquinolone to provide broader antimicrobial coverage.[18] Gentamycin dosage should be calculated at 5 mg/kg.[3] The gentamycin dosage for a morbidly obese patient should be calculated using a patient's ideal weight in addition to 40% of the excess weight.[3] The recommended timing of antibiotics is within 60 minutes of incision time, with the exception of vancomycin described previously. This allows the drug to reach the tissue at a level that effectively inhibits the potential contaminant organism during the initial surgical incisions.[3] Some evidence suggests the optimal window is within 0 to 30 minutes prior to incision.[3] The duration of prophylactic antibiotics should not extend beyond 24 hours after surgery end time.[3,18] Prolonged duration of prophylactic antibiotics does not increase efficacy in preventing SSIs and increases the potential for development of multi-drug resistant organisms and clostridium difficile infection.

Although the appropriate selection of antibiotic agents for CABG and the appropriate dosages are easily built into electronic order sets, the timing of the preoperative antibiotic with skin incision requires teamwork and coordination by anesthesia, pharmacy, surgeons, and nurses. Electronic alerts can remind clinicians to redose cefazolin in the operating room if needed. The medication administration process in the electronic medical record enables the nurse to be alerted prior to administering a prophylactic antibiotic past the recommended duration time. A notice to the pharmacist that the patient is receiving prophylactic antibiotics after surgery may help to avoid the rescheduling of doses to inadvertently extend past the recommended duration. These alerts can help hardwire evidence-based care through creating a redundant system for clinicians. See **Figs. 1** and **2** for examples of hardwiring evidence-based prophylactic antibiotic prescribing.

Preoperative Nasal Decolonization with Mupirocin

Mupirocin administration is recognized as an effective strategy to decrease SSI by decolonizing patients who are intranasal carriers of MRSA when used in combination with prophylactic antibiotics.[18] Screening patients for MRSA can present a significant cost burden to an organization, especially where the appropriate testing equipment is not already available. Due to this expense, some organizations have prescribed mupirocin to all patients undergoing high-risk procedures, regardless of screening and/or

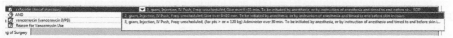

Fig. 1. Weight-based dosing of cefazolin in order set.

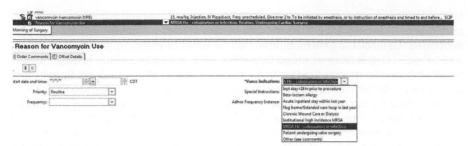

Fig. 2. Documentation of high-risk indications for ordering vancomycin as prophylactic antibiotic.

known colonization.[19] The risk associated with the administration of mupirocin to all patients, regardless of colonization status or risk of SSI, is the development of mupirocin-resistant microorganisms.[3,18] Miller and colleagues[20] documented the accelerated development of mupirocin-resistant MRSA within one organization from 2.7% in 1990 to 65% in 1993 after widespread use of mupirocin ointment for infection control. The 2014 update to "Strategies to Prevent Surgical Site Infections in Acute Care Hospitals" lists mupirocin as a "special approach for preventing SSI" to be used in addition to standard SSI prevention interventions in the setting of unacceptably high SSI rates.[3] When mupirocin is used, it is prescribed for intranasal administration twice daily for 5 days preoperatively.[18] Patient education is necessary to achieve uniform adherence to this regimen.

Glycemic Control

Use of a continuous intravenous insulin infusion protocol is recommended in the 2011 American College of Cardiology Foundation and American Heart Association CABG guidelines to keep blood glucose (BG) less than 180 mg/dL.[19] More recently, a meta-analysis published in 2015 by Boreland and colleagues[9] supports the use of an insulin protocol to maintain BG less than 200 mg/dL. This meta-analysis included 4 randomized controlled trials and 7 cohort studies that reported on the outcome of SSI in diabetic patients. SSIs occurred in 59 of the 5994 patients who received a continuous insulin infusion to maintain BG less than 200 mg/dL compared with 111 postoperative infections among the 3369 patients in the control group who did not receive a continuous insulin infusion. The meta-analysis found the continuous insulin infusion group lowered the rate of postoperative infections by an odds ratio of 0.37 (95% CI, 0.27–0.52; $P<.00001$).[9] A prospective descriptive study published in 2015 attempted to associate outcomes after cardiac surgery with the time the patient spent within target BG range (BG approximately 108–146 mg/dL).[21] The study included 227 patients, including 100 patients with diabetes and 127 patients without diabetes. The patients were divided into 2 groups: group 1 included those who were within target range greater than 80% of the time during the insulin infusion, and group 2 included those who were within target range less than 80% of the time during the insulin infusion. Group 1 had significantly less SSIs. In group 1, 3 of 146 patients (2.1%) developed a SSI versus 7 of 81 patients (8.6%) in group 2 ($P = .05$). Group 2 also had significantly higher length of stay in the ICU ($P = .04$) and in the hospital ($P = .03$), duration of mechanical ventilation ($P = .03$), and incidence of postoperative atrial fibrillation ($P = .04$) compared with group 1.[21]

Although the recent Surgical Care Improvement Project quality measures called for controlling postoperative glucose levels within 18 to 24 hours after surgery, clinicians who have worked to achieve glycemic control in these patients are acutely aware that preoperative planning and aggressive control strategies during the intraoperative period are required to achieve postoperative control. The continuous insulin infusion is another SSI prevention strategy that must be a collaborative effort between the surgeon, perfusionist, and anesthesia clinicians in the operating room. This collaboration can be further supported by the interprofessional SSI prevention team and requires ongoing education and feedback to be successful in achieving optimal glycemic control throughout the postoperative period. Clinical pharmacists are invaluable in helping the team transition patients from a continuous insulin infusion to a subcutaneous insulin regimen when indicated. Patients frequently require greater insulin dosages in the immediate postoperative period, and the clinical pharmacist can serve as a consultant to the hospitalist or surgeon during this transition. Another complicating factor when determining the dose for transition of insulin from intravenous infusion to the subcutaneous route is poor preoperative glycemic control, particularly in the setting of incomplete adherence to the insulin regimen at home. This makes determination of a postoperative insulin regimen difficult. The clinical pharmacist can provide expertise, monitor the patient's response, and facilitate revision of the plan when necessary. Certified diabetes educators and licensed dietitians are also critical team members for patients with suboptimal glycemic control based on preoperative hemoglobin A_{1c} levels and history or self-report. For these patients, endocrinologists are best consulted preoperatively to revise the postoperative glycemic control regimen immediately after the insulin infusion and coordinate an optimal discharge transition plan.

Surgical Technique

There are some basic SSI prevention strategies related to surgical technique, such as minimizing the use of electrocautery and avoiding excessive manipulation of tissue and hematoma formation whenever possible.[5,15] There are other surgical techniques whose effectiveness in SSI prevention have not been confirmed, such as the use of antiseptic impregnated sutures and gentamycin-collagen sponges.[3]

Incision Care and Postoperative Bathing

Surgical incisions should be covered in the operating room with sterile dressings and should remain covered for 24 to 48 hours[15] to allow for complete epithelialization of the wound. Bath basins should not be reused, due to findings from a multicenter study by Johnson and colleagues[22] that revealed bacterial growth in 98% of 92 bath basins sampled from 3 ICUs. Although not supported by SSI prevention guidelines, some ICUs have implemented daily bathing of patients with CHG. SSI prevention guidelines are not prescriptive regarding bathing and incision care after removal of the dressing 48 hours after surgery end time.[3,15] A sample incision care protocol consistent with those published in performance improvement cohort studies is presented in **Fig. 3**.

THE INTERPROFESSIONAL TEAM AS A CRITICAL STRUCTURE FOR DECREASING SURGICAL SITE INFECTION

Prevention of SSI in CABG patients requires the vigilance of numerous interprofessional team members caring for CABG patients, from the preoperative staff interacting with the patient through the intraoperative period, critical and progressive care, and postdischarge clinicians (**Box 2**). In addition to the individual clinicians providing care for patients undergoing CABG, an important group of clinicians in critiquing,

Operating Room

Chest tube dressing and sternal incision dressing will be taped separately, so the chest tube dressings can be removed without disturbing the sternal wound dressing.

Leg incisions will be dressed with sterile dressings to prevent contamination.

Intensive Care Unit

The ICU admit nurse will label the dressings with date and end time from surgery.

Dressings will remain on for 48 h post-op.

⇒ If wound drainage is noted, dressings can be reinforced as needed.

⇒ If patient remains intubated at 48 h, dressing will be maintained on sternal wound to prevent contamination from respiratory secretions.

Stepdown Unit

48 h Post-Op: Dressings are removed.

Incisions are left open to air as long as they are well-approximated without drainage.

If any incision is draining and/or is not well approximated when removed at 48 h:

⇒ Clean incisions with sterile saline

⇒ Cover with sterile dressing after cleaned and change sterile dressing daily

⇒ Consult wound care nurse to check wound and recommend further treatment

⇒ Notify CVT surgeon if not already aware

Daily bath with soap and water. Wash incisions first with clean washcloth.

If pacer wires are out, encourage showering on post-op Day 4,

and instruct the patient to wash incision areas first with clean washcloth.

Fig. 3. Incision care protocol.

implementing, and evaluating the effectiveness of SSI prevention strategies is the interprofessional SSI prevention team. Since the "Guideline for Prevention of Surgical Site Infection" was published in 1999,[15] other guidelines have been published by various professional organizations, performance improvement organizations, and experts.[3,5,18,19,23] These SSI guidelines and prevention toolkits require the expertise of many disciplines and specialties for an effective review and gap analysis of current practices within an organization. Evaluation of new practices is further complicated by the recent tendency to implement "bundles" of interventions and publish SSI outcomes. This could be partially due to increased regulation and public reporting of SSI

Box 2
Interprofessional roles to consider for inclusion in surgical site infection prevention team

- Infection Preventionist
- Surgery Circulating Nurse and Leader
- Surgery Concurrent Review Nurse
- Surgeon
- Nurse Educator
- Nurse from acute care and critical care
- Pharmacist
- Anesthesiologist
- Certified Registered Nurse Anesthetist
- Endocrinologist
- Licensed Dietician
- Certified Diabetes Educator
- Preoperative Assessment and Education Nurse
- Surgery Informatics Nurse
- Clinical Nurse Specialist
- Chief Nursing Officer
- Chief Medical Officer

---

data, which may cause organizations to feel pressure to implement multiple strategies at once to prevent SSIs. This bundle strategy makes it more difficult to evaluate the effectiveness of the individual SSI prevention interventions included in the bundle. An interprofessional team that uses its collective expertise to interpret evidence and collaborates to facilitate adoption of evidence-based strategies for prevention of SSI in patients undergoing CABG is essential.[3,24]

Role of the Surgery Concurrent Review Nurse in Preventing Surgical Site Infection

The 2014 update to the "Strategies to Prevent Surgical Site Infections in Acute Care Hospitals"[3] recommends mitigating modifiable risk factors within the operating room environment. The surgery concurrent review nurse is in a unique position to provide education to operating room staff regarding evidence-based practices to prevent SSI. The surgery concurrent review nurse observes the surgical site skin preparation, aseptic technique, proper attire, and hand hygiene by the surgeon and other members of the surgical team. The surgery concurrent review nurse is able to monitor and help minimize traffic in operating rooms. This nurse can coordinate with the appropriate departments to achieve air handling, sterilization, equipment, and environmental cleaning standards. Peer feedback can be given during real-time audits, and concurrent review can be triggered as patients are scheduled for surgery. The surgery concurrent review nurse uses skilled communication to collaborate with surgical teams in the operating room, nurses and staff on hospital units, and the organization's SSI prevention team. Through these collaborative relationships, the organization can strategically identify and remove barriers to implementing evidence-based SSI prevention strategies and support clinicians with education and feedback.

Role of the Postoperative Nurses in Evaluating Patient Outcomes Related to Surgical Site Infection

Nurses caring for the postoperative CABG patient can easily evaluate daily outcomes related to SSI prevention in a structured format, such as a clinical pathway (**Fig. 4**). Clinical pathways for CABG in the electronic medical record can pull in previously documented information to make outcome evaluation less time-consuming for nurses. Some SSI prevention strategies and surveillance that may be included in a clinical pathway include:

- Incision site surveillance and care
- Temperature monitoring and reporting of fever
- Assessment of patient's overall oxygenation status through oxygen saturation as measured by pulse oximetry monitoring
- Achievement of glycemic control goals
- Prompts to remind nurses and cardiac rehabilitation clinicians to teach patients and caregivers about signs and symptoms to observe for after discharge and how to report them

Ongoing Evaluation of New Evidence-Based Practices with an Interprofessional Team Approach

One of the roles of the interprofessional SSI prevention team is to evaluate newly published evidence-based practices for appropriateness within an organization. One such recent practice is the application of povidone-iodine ointment as a nasal antiseptic to suppress microbial activity for the duration of surgery in patients colonized with *S aureus*. In a randomized study comparing intranasal application of mupirocin with intranasal application of povidone-iodine in patients undergoing arthroplasty or spine surgery, Phillips and colleagues[25] demonstrated no significant differences in deep *S aureus* SSI or deep SSI caused by any pathogen. All patients used CHG wipes on the morning of surgery. All patients had verbal and written instructions and access to 24/7 telephonic support in case of study-related treatment questions. Mupirocin patients used the 2% intranasal preparation according to instructions twice daily for 5 days prior to surgery. Povidone-iodine patients completed two 30-second applications into each nostril within 2 hours of surgical incision. Interprofessional team members, such as infection control preventionists, pharmacists, nurses, physicians, leaders, and educators, can provide unique perspectives in evaluating this novel SSI prevention strategy.

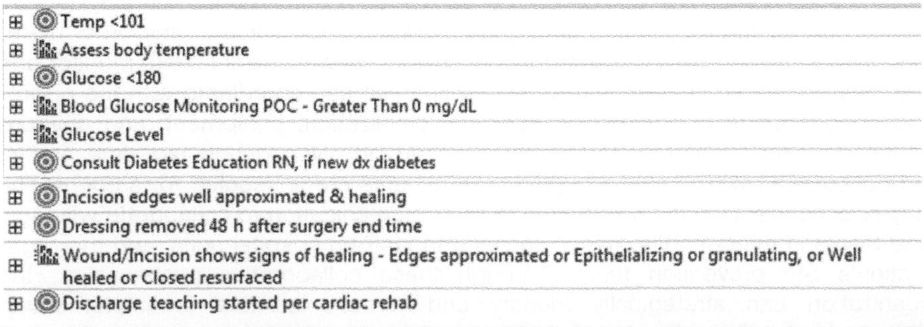

⊞ ◎	Temp <101
⊞ ▦	Assess body temperature
⊞ ◎	Glucose <180
⊞ ▦	Blood Glucose Monitoring POC - Greater Than 0 mg/dL
⊞ ▦	Glucose Level
⊞ ◎	Consult Diabetes Education RN, if new dx diabetes
⊞ ◎	Incision edges well approximated & healing
⊞ ◎	Dressing removed 48 h after surgery end time
⊞ ▦	Wound/Incision shows signs of healing - Edges approximated or Epithelializing or granulating, or Well healed or Closed resurfaced
⊞ ◎	Discharge teaching started per cardiac rehab

Fig. 4. SSI prevention outcomes evaluated using CABG clinical pathway. Dx, diagnosis; POC, point of care.

Interprofessional Analysis of Patient Data and Trends to Direct Education and Interventions

Root cause analysis and/or failure modes and effects analysis may be conducted to analyze infections that occur and lapses in SSI prevention strategies that are identified.[3] Tools and instructions have been published in various toolkits that can be used for this purpose by the SSI prevention team.[3,4,23] Data, trends, and solutions identified by a interprofessional SSI prevention team must be shared with all frontline clinicians when discovered. Clinicians who regularly provide care to these patients can provide insight, identify barriers, help develop education, and effectively incorporate any changes into practice.[3]

Practice Gap Analysis Using Newly Published Guidelines

An SSI prevention team is the ideal group to conduct a gap analysis when new SSI prevention guidelines, toolkits, or meta-analyses are published. The team should be supported by administration and performance improvement experts capable of facilitating rapid-cycle change until a superior process can be hardwired into clinicians' workflow. Multiple forms of communication are preferred for all members of the SSI prevention team to report data, trends, changes in practice, and new evidence-based initiatives.[24] For example, Stoodley and colleagues[26] describe decreasing SSIs after cardiac surgery through standardizing incision care. A strategy used by this team was a pretest of nurses caring for the cardiac surgery patients. This helped focus education on SSI prevention, detection, and mitigation strategies. The team disseminated information regarding the new evidence-based dressing changes and other SSI prevention education through various formats, including skills stations, educational programs, best-practice champions, visual cues/reminders on the units, one-on-one coaching, and regular surveillance by a nurse practitioner to increase compliance with the protocol. The nurses' post-test scores were significantly higher on 8 of 12 questions, and the program has resulted in progressive and sustained annual decreases in the SSI rate. The team plans to monitor sternal wound care indefinitely and is developing ongoing education and mentoring programs, including orientation materials and unit-based protocol books.[26]

Prevention of SSI in patients undergoing CABG surgery requires continual evaluation of evidence and individual patient and organizational outcomes using an interprofessional team approach. Hardwiring of standards and processes through electronic order sets, prompts, protocols, and clinical pathways aids in SSI prevention strategies when supported by clinician input, education, and feedback. Some strategies are less amenable to hardwiring, and require more structured surveillance with ongoing feedback and action plans when opportunities for improvement are identified. An interprofessional team approach by clinicians caring for patients undergoing CABG surgery throughout the continuum of care is essential for SSI prevention.

ACKNOWLEDGMENTS

The authors would like to thank Sally Fenerty, BSL, hospital librarian, for her invaluable assistance and expertise in obtaining literature for this review and Michelle Atzenhoffer, BSN, RN, CIC; Christina Hoppe, BSN, RN-BC; Marisa Morton, BSN, RN, PCCN; Shavonne Williams, MN, APRN, ACNS-BC, CCRN; and Bridget Boogaerts, BSN, RN-BC, ONC, CRRN, PCCN for reviewing the article. The authors also wish to recognize their esteemed colleagues who implement SSI prevention measures while providing excellent care to the cardiac surgery patient population every day.

REFERENCES

1. Musallam E. The predictors of surgical site infection post cardiac surgery: a systematic review. J Vasc Nurs 2014;32(3):105–18.
2. Surgical Site Infection (SSI) Event. CDC Web site. Available at: http://www.cdc.gov/nhsn/PDFs/pscManual/9pscSSIcurrent.pdf. Accessed April 25, 2016.
3. Anderson DJ, Podgorny K, Berrios-Torres SI, et al. Strategies to prevent surgical site infections in acute care hospitals: 2014 update. Infect Control Hosp Epidemiol 2014;35(6):605–27.
4. National and states healthcare associated infections progress report. CDC Web site. Available at: http://www.cdc.gov/HAI/pdfs/progress-report/hai-progress-report.pdf. Accessed April 25, 2016.
5. Kohut K. APIC guide for the prevention of Mediastinitis surgical site infection following cardiac surgery. The APIC Web site. Available at: http://apic.org/Resource_/EliminationGuideForm/a994706c-8e6c-4807-b89a-6a7e6fb863dd/File/APIC-Mediastinitis-Elimination-Guide.pdf. Accessed April 20, 2016.
6. Greco G, Shi W, Michler RE, et al. Costs associated with health care-associated infections in cardiac surgery. J Am Coll Cardiol 2015;65(1):15–23.
7. Anthony A, Sendelbach S. Postoperative complications of coronary artery bypass grafting surgery. Crit Care Nurs Clin North Am 2007;19(4):403–15.
8. Redzek A, Mironicki M, Gvozdenovic A, et al. Predictors for hospital readmission after cardiac surgery. J Card Surg 2015;30:1–6.
9. Boreland L, Scott-Hudson M, Hetherington K, et al. The effectiveness of tight glycemic control on decreasing surgical site infections and readmission rates in adult patients with diabetes undergoing cardiac surgery: a systematic review. Heart Lung 2015;44:430–40.
10. National action plan to prevent health care-associated infections: road map to elimination. Office of Disease Prevention and Health Promotion Web site. Available at: http://health.gov/hcq/pdfs/HAI-Targets.pdf. Accessed April 25, 2016.
11. Kubota H, Miyata H, Motomura N, et al. Deep sternal wound infection after cardiac surgery. J Cardiothorac Surg 2013;8:132–7.
12. Bryan CS, Yarbrough WM. Preventing deep wound infection after coronary artery bypass grafting. Tex Heart Inst J 2013;40(2):125–39.
13. Kayani WT, Bandeali SJ, Lee VV, et al. Association between statins and infections after coronary artery bypass grafting. Int J Cardiol 2013;168:117–20.
14. Mauermann WJ, Sampathkumar P, Thompson RL. Sternal wound infections. Best Pract Res Clin Anaesthesiol 2008;22(3):423–36.
15. Mangram AJ, Horan TC, Pearson ML, et al. Guideline for prevention of surgical site infection. Infect Control Hosp Epidemiol 1999;20(4):250–78.
16. Webster J, Osborne S. Preoperative bathing or showering with skin antiseptics to prevent surgical site infection. Cochrane Database Syst Rev 2015;(2):CD004985.
17. Boyce JM, Pittet D, Healthcare Infection Control Practices Advisory Committee, HICPAC/SHEA/APIC/IDSA Hand Hygiene Task Force. Guideline for hand hygiene in health-care settings. Recommendations of the Healthcare Infection Control Practices Advisory Committee and the HICPAC/SHEA/APIC/IDSA hand hygiene task force. society for healthcare epidemiology of America/Association for Professionals in Infection Control/Infectious diseases society of America. MMWR Recomm Rep 2002;51(RR-16):1–45.
18. Bratzler DW, Dellinger EP, Olsen KM, et al. Clinical practice guidelines for antimicrobial prophylaxis in surgery. Am J Health Syst Pharm 2013;70:195–283.

19. Hills LD, Smith PK, Anderson JL, et al. ACCF/AHA guideline for coronary artery bypass graft surgery: executive summary. Circulation 2011;124:2610–42.
20. Miller MA, Dascal A, Portnoy J, et al. Development of Mupirocin resistance among methicillin-resistant staphylococcus aureus after widespread use of nasal Mupirocin ointment. Infect Control Hosp Epidemiol 1996;17(12):811–3.
21. Omar AS, Salama A, Allam M, et al. Association of time in blood glucose range with outcomes following cardiac surgery. BMC Anesthesiol 2015;15:14–21.
22. Johnson D, Lineweaver L, Maze L. Patients' bath basins as potential sources of infection: a multicenter sampling study. Am J Crit Care 2009;18:31–40.
23. How-to guide: prevent surgical site infections. Institute for Healthcare Improvement Web site. 2012. Available at: www.ihi.org. Accessed April 25, 2016.
24. Travis J, Carr JB, Saylor D, et al. Coronary artery bypass graft surgery: surgical site infection prevention. J Healthc Qual 2009;31(4):16–23.
25. Phillips M, Rosenberg A, Shopsin B, et al. Preventing surgical site infections: a randomized, open-label trial of nasal mupirocin ointment and nasal povidone iodine solution. Infect Control Hosp Epidemiol 2014;35(7):826–32.
26. Stoodley L, Lillington L, Ansryan L, et al. Sternal wound care to prevent infections in adult cardiac surgery patients. Crit Care Nurs Q 2012;35(1):76–84.

Management of Sepsis in Patients with Pulmonary Arterial Hypertension in the Intensive Care Unit

Todd M. Tartavoulle, DNS, APRN, CNS-BC

KEYWORDS

- Pulmonary arterial hypertension • Sepsis • Right ventricular failure • Cardiac output

KEY POINTS

- Sepsis is an inflammatory process that results in increased capillary membrane permeability and vasodilation.
- Hemodynamic changes that occur in sepsis include a decrease in systemic vascular resistance (SVR) that must be compensated by an increase in cardiac output (CO).
- In pulmonary arterial hypertension (PAH), there is an increase in right ventricular end diastolic pressure and a decrease in CO.
- Management of septic shock in PAH is complex.
- Goals of therapy include maintaining tissue perfusion and eradicating the cause.

Sepsis begins with an inflammatory process that results in increased capillary membrane permeability and vasodilation. Proinflammatory and anti-inflammatory mechanisms are activated and contribute to a cascade of endothelial injury, global tissue hypoxia, and formation of microthrombi. Patients with sepsis experience a decrease in intravascular volume and a fall in SVR that must be compensated for by an increase in CO. In patients diagnosed with PAH, the ability to suddenly increase CO to meet increased metabolic demands may be severely limited. Patients with increased pulmonary artery pressures in the setting of sepsis may experience rapid deterioration of right ventricular function, hemodynamic instability, and death.[1–4] As a result, the management of septic shock in PAH patients in the intensive care unit can be extremely challenging.

The pulmonary vasculature contains arteries and arterioles that branch in the lungs to create a dense capillary bed to advance blood flow. The pulmonary capillary bed is

The author has nothing to disclose.
School of Nursing, Louisiana State University Health Sciences Center, 1900 Gravier Street, New Orleans, LA 70112, USA
E-mail address: TTARTA@LSUHSC.EDU

0899-5885/17/© 2016 Elsevier Inc. All rights reserved.
ccnursing.theclinics.com

a high-volume, low-pressure, low-resistance system and is highly vascularized as blood is delivered to and taken away by arterial and venous circulations, respectively. Despite generating essentially the same CO, the vascular bed through which the right and left ventricles pump is very different. The pulmonary vascular resistance (PVR), through which the right ventricle must pump against, is remarkably low (less than 150 dynes/s/cm^5/m^2) and the SVR through which the left ventricle must pump against is considerably higher (800–1200 dynes/s/cm^5/m^2). In healthy individuals, the arterioles are able to dilate in times of increased metabolic demand. During exercise, the CO may increase by 4-fold above baseline with a minimal increase in pulmonary artery pressure and reduction in PVR.[3,5]

In PAH, there is an increase in pulmonary artery resistance and right ventricular failure as a result of smooth cell proliferation in the intima causing a thickening of the arteriole walls with progressive vascular narrowing.[6,7] This leads to elevated PVR and increased right ventricular end-diastolic pressure. As right ventricular end-diastolic pressure rises and exceeds left ventricular end-diastolic pressure, the interventricular septum shifts toward the left ventricle, decreasing left ventricular compliance, resulting in decreased left ventricular CO. The ability of filling pressures of the right ventricle to affect filling pressures of the left ventricle via the interventricular septum is referred to as ventricular interdependence. Ventricular interdependence represents a challenge to fluid management in PAH patients who are in septic shock.[3]

MANAGEMENT OF SEPSIS IN PULMONARY ARTERIAL HYPERTENSION

Patients with PAH presenting with septic shock have inadequate perfusion of tissues and lack adequate oxygen delivery to organs resulting in lactic acidosis, multiorgan failure and possibly death. Septic shock must be treated immediately to minimize the risk for multiple organ failure and death. The need for aggressive management of infectious complications in PAH patients with septic shock is warranted because sepsis at any time in an intensive care unit is a strong predictor of death.[8]

Management of septic shock in PAH is complex and requires expertise. Goals of therapy include maintaining adequate tissue perfusion by increasing intravascular volume and increasing CO while eradicating the cause. In patients with PAH, goal-directed therapy focuses on augmenting right ventricular function while decreasing PVR. Strategies to maximize right ventricular function include optimizing right ventricular preload, improving right ventricular contractility, and reducing right ventricular afterload, which is achieved by lessening PVR. In PAH, an acute reduction in PVR is problematic due to the relatively fixed nature of the pulmonary vascular disease. Treatment strategies are directed at optimizing right ventricular function and limiting increases in PVR in response to metabolic derangements caused by sepsis or vasopressors administered during resuscitation.[3,7,9]

RIGHT VENTRICULAR PRELOAD

Treatment of septic shock in PAH patients should be initiated as quickly as possible with proper fluid management. Once an organism invades a host, an inflammatory response is initiated to restore homeostasis. Cytokines are released and damage endothelial cells that line blood vessels resulting in profound vasodilation and increased capillary permeability. A decrease in intravascular volume and venous vascular tone lowers central venous pressure (CVP).[1,3,10]

To maintain CO in acute right ventricular decompensation in septic shock, establishing adequate right-sided filling pressure is essential. Therefore, early goal-directed therapy includes initiation of volume resuscitation if CVP is low. Fluid management is often difficult in septic shock patients with PAH because right ventricular failure may occur with an increase in right ventricular afterload. Volume loading may result in interventricular septal displacement toward the left ventricle, impairing left ventricular diastolic filling. In this case, intravascular volume may need to be decreased. Careful measuring and monitoring of CVP are important to guide volume resuscitation.[3]

Diagnostic tests can be performed to evaluate volume status. Transthoracic echocardiography reveals right ventricular dilation with impingement on left ventricle with volume overload. This suggests further reduction in preload is necessary. Assessment of the inferior vena caval filling via ultrasound is another diagnostic assessment to evaluate right ventricular preload. If these assessments of right ventricular function and preload are inadequate, placement of a pulmonary artery catheter may be necessary.[3]

If right ventricular preload is elevated, diuresis or dialysis therapy should be initiated to reduce CVP and subsequently increase CO. CO can be assessed by either central venous oxygen saturation ($Scvo_2$) or mixed venous oxygen saturation (Svo_2) and systemic perfusion. An $Scvo_2$ between 65% and 85% and an Svo_2 between 60% and 80% indicate an adequate balance between oxygen supply and demand. A lower $Scvo_2$ or Svo_2 in the setting of normal arterial oxygenation may indicate a diminished CO.[3,11]

A negative fluid balance may be necessary before any improvement in right ventricular function occurs. At the same time, hypovolemia may have detrimental effects because right ventricular output is dependent on adequate right ventricular filling when PVR is high.[12]

Fluid management in PAH patients with septic shock is often difficult because both hypovolemia and hypervolemia can have adverse effects on cardiac function and organ perfusion. Maintenance of an adequate CO in the septic PAH patient is critically important. Right ventricular failure leading to an inadequate CO may result from poor or excess preload or an elevated PVR due to deteriorating pulmonary hypertension. Even with an adequate preload and a reduction in PVR, the ability of the right ventricle to distribute an effective CO may be reduced. In septic shock, acid/base imbalances and inflammatory cytokines may cause a decrease in myocardial contractile forces, decrease in coronary artery perfusion, and an increase in preload. This results in overstretching of the right ventricular free wall, reduction in contractility, and decreased CO.[10]

VASOPRESSORS

Right ventricular failure with low CO and profound hypotension in PAH patients with septic shock is difficult to treat and may require a vasopressor to raise mean arterial pressure (MAP) and CO. The ideal pharmacologic therapy should raise MAP and increase right ventricular contractility without raising right ventricular afterload (PVR). Norepinephrine is a vasoconstrictor agent and stimulates α_1- and β_1-adrenergic receptors. Stimulation of α_1-receptors causes vasoconstriction resulting in adequate systemic blood pressure and coronary artery perfusion, required to maintain cardiac function. In animal studies, norepinephrine's β_1 effects include increased contractility with an improvement in pulmonary artery/right ventricular coupling in right ventricular failure.[3,13–15]

Phenylephrine, a pure α_1-receptor agonist, is a powerful arterial vasoconstrictor that augments right coronary artery perfusion. Phenylephrine increases right ventricular afterload (PVR) and decreases CO, however, thus worsening right ventricular preload in PAH patients. The myocytes of the right ventricular free wall become overstretched and CO decreases. A potential side effect of phenylephrine is reflex bradycardia, which further decreases CO.[3,10,12]

Epinephrine is a potent mixed α-adrenergic and β-adrenergic agonist.

Epinephrine has mixed properties and increases both mean arterial BP by vasoconstriction (α-adrenergic effect) and CO (β-adrenergic effect).[16]

Vasopressin has systemic vasoconstrictive properties by activating V1 receptors on vascular smooth muscle cells.[8] Vasopressin stimulates endothelial nitric oxide (NO) causing selective pulmonary vasodilation at low doses (0.01–0.03 U/min). At higher doses, vasopressin increases mean pulmonary arterial pressure (MPAP) and PVR, causes coronary artery vasoconstriction, and reduces CO.[16]

Norepinephrine is the preferred agent to treat persistent hypotension in PAH patients who are in septic shock. Norepinephrine raises, SVR, which was lowered initially due to the systemic infection.[3]

INOTROPES

The goal of inotropes in PAH patients with septic shock is to augment CO. Dobutamine acts primarily on β_1-adrenergic receptors to increase contractility and may act on β_2-adrenergic receptors to reduce right and left ventricular afterload.[8] In animal studies, dobutamine at low doses (5–10 $\mu g/kg^{-1}/min^{-1}$) significantly decreased PVR while slightly increasing CO. Higher doses should be avoided because the risk of β_2-mediated vasodilation, hypotension, and significant tachycardia increases.[3,12,13,17]

Dopamine is a dose-dependent adrenergic and dopaminergic agonist that raises MAP and CO. Dopamine activates dopaminergic receptors at low doses (less than 5 $\mu g/kg^{-1}/min^{-1}$), β_1-receptors at doses of 5 $\mu g/kg^{-1}/min^{-1}$ to 10 $\mu g/kg^{-1}/min^{-1}$, and α_1-receptors at doses greater than 10 $\mu g/kg^{-1}/min^{-1}$. Increases in CO without subsequent increases in PVR generally occur in doses less than 16 $\mu g/kg^{-1}/min^{-1}$.[3,12,13] Dopamine may cause significant tachycardia that may decrease left ventricular preload and worsen demand ischemia. Tachycardia reduces diastolic filling time causing adverse effects in patients with PAH.[10]

Milrinone, a PDE type 3, does not possess chronotropic properties and may be preferable. This drug exhibits direct inotropic effects by inhibition of PDE leading to elevated levels of endogenous cyclic adenosine monophosphate and indirectly increases CO by reducing PVR.[3,12]

Inotropes improve right ventricular contractility; however, adverse side effects include tachyarrhythmias and a drop in SVR, making their use in septic shock controversial. Inotropes should be considered in PAH patients with sepsis only after abnormalities in right ventricular preload and contractility have been corrected and inadequate oxygen delivery remains as evidence by decreasing $Scvo_2$ or Svo_2.[3]

PULMONARY VASCULAR RESISTANCE

In PAH patients, PVR is elevated due to smooth cell proliferation in the intima causing thickening and clogging of the arteriole walls. The injured area inside the arterioles forms plexiform lesions, which clog the insides of the arterioles and cause scar formation of the intima and media. As a result of this pathophysiologic process, it can be difficult if not impossible to acutely lower PVR. Patients with PAH may have increased muscularization of proximal pulmonary vessels and some are capable of vasoconstriction; therefore, it is vital to avert any factors that may increase PVR while at the same time attempting to administer pharmacologic agents to cause pulmonary artery vasodilation.[3]

In septic shock, an increase in PVR can occur as a result of hypoxic pulmonary vasoconstriction, overdistension of alveoli at high lung volume from mechanical ventilation, thrombosis in situ in the pulmonary circulation, an increase in the release of vasoactive factors (endothelin and thrombosis), and release of endotoxin, which suppresses NO synthesis. These factors can contribute to increase PVR during sepsis and every attempt should be made to lower PVR by reversing any of these factors before initiating pulmonary vasodilation.[3]

Pharmacologic treatment involves using medications that target cellular pathways that are abnormally regulated in PAH (**Table 1**). These drugs restore the vasodilator effects, prevent overgrowth of cells, and have been shown to improve functional capacity, reduce PVR, and increase CO. The ability of these drugs to improve pulmonary hemodynamics in PAH patients with sepsis has not been studied. Despite a lack of clinical efficacy, administration of PAH specific drugs may be necessary to reduce PVR and increase CO. Although these drugs target the pulmonary vasculature and cause pulmonary vasorelaxation, they may also have significant effects on the systemic circulation and cause hypotension. Other adverse effects include worsening of gas exchange by blunting hypoxic pulmonary vasoconstriction, thereby causing ventilation-perfusion mismatch.[18]

Inhaled agents, by virtue of their route, have the potential advantage of selective delivery to the pulmonary circulation with less systemic effects. Inhaled NO is a potent vasodilator of the pulmonary circulation with a rapid onset of action and an extremely short half-life. For this reason, inhaled NO is an optimal medication for septic shock PAH patients with right ventricular dysfunction. NO induces soluble guanylate cyclase to increase cyclic guanosine monophosphate (cGMP). As a result, intracellular calcium levels are reduced, causing vasodilation in the precapillary resistance arterioles. Inhaled NO prevents an increase in the alveolar to arterial gradient in well ventilated lungs and can raise oxygen levels by decreasing intrapulmonary shunt. Although the use of inhaled NO in septic PAH patients has not been studied, patients with acute respiratory distress syndrome with PAH have had significant decreases in MPAP and PVR and increases in right ventricular ejection fraction and end-diastolic volume.[3,12,19]

Prostanoids, such as epoprostenol, trepostinil, and iloprost, may be used to treat PAH and can be administered via inhalation. These 3 medications may be a reasonable alternative if inhaled NO is not available. Epoprostenol dilates blood vessels, prevents platelets from clumping together and increases CO. Treprostinil's mechanism of action produces pulmonary vasodilation thereby reducing right and left ventricular

Table 1
Summary of targeted medication therapy used to treat pulmonary arterial hypertension

Class of Medication	Name	Route of Administration	Terminal Half-Life
Prostanoids	Iloprost	Inhaled	20–30 min
	Treprostinil	IV, subcutaneous Inhaled	4 h
	Epoprostenol	IV	<6 min
Endothelin receptor antagonists	Ambrisentan	Oral	15 h
	Bosentan	Oral	5 h
	Macitentan	Oral	14–18 h
PDE-5 inhibitors	Sildenafil	Oral, IV	4 h orally
	Tadalafil	Oral	17.5 h
Soluble guanylate cyclase stimulator	Riociguat	Oral	7–12 h

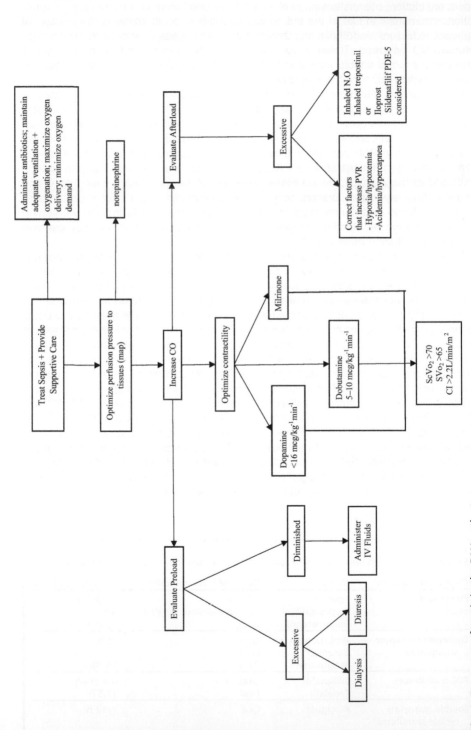

Fig. 1. Treatment of sepsis in the PAH patient.

afterload with an increase in CO. Iloprost can also be inhaled via nebulizer and its effects are confined to the lungs, so adverse effects are minimal.[3,8,12]

Phosphodiesterase (PDE) type 5 (PDE-5) inhibitors, function by inhibiting cGMP-specific PDE-5. By inhibiting metabolism of PDE-5, cGMP is not broken down and relaxation of pulmonary blood vessels occurs. PDE-5 inhibitors have improved contractility in the setting of right ventricular hypertrophy in animal studies of pulmonary hypertension.[3,20] Little is known about their use in critical illness and caution should be used in PAH patients in septic shock because of their potential systemic hypotensive effects and prolonged half-life. Sildenafil does have a shorter half-life than tadalafil and should be drug of choice if a PDE-5 inhibitor is considered. Sildenafil is available both intravenously (IV) and orally.[21]

Endothelin receptor antagonists (bosentan and ambrisentan) and soluble guanylate cyclase stimulator (riociguat) are other currently available pulmonary vasodilators that are used in the management of PAH. Endothelin receptor antagonists prevent cell growth in the arteries by preventing endothelin from activating receptors. This class of drugs has less acute effects on pulmonary hemodynamics and may affect liver function and the metabolism of other medications. Riociguat, a soluble guanylate cyclase stimulator, causes the blood vessels in the pulmonary vasculature to relax and widen. Riociguat may cause systemic hypotension especially in a septic condition.[20]

Calcium channel blockers affect the electrical system of the heart and can slow down fast heart rates. Because of their negative inotropic effects, calcium channel blockers should not be used.[3,22] See **Fig. 1** for a graphic approach in the treatment of sepsis in PAH patients.

MECHANICAL VENTILATION

Mechanical ventilation may be warranted in septic shock PAH patients who develop respiratory failure as a result of acute respiratory distress syndrome. Mechanical ventilation can increase lung volume and decrease functional residual capacity, which increases PVR and right ventricular afterload. In PAH patients with poor right ventricular output, hyperinflated lungs and either adequate or excessive positive end-expiratory pressure can fatally reduce CO. Prior research results suggest optimal ventilator management in PAH patients should include low tidal volumes and relatively low positive end-expiratory pressure. This ventilation strategy is similar to ventilator management of the acute respiratory distress syndrome patient, but extreme efforts should be taken to avoid permissive hypercapnia. Permissive hypercapnia can increase PVR and MPAP and further diminish CO. Mechanical ventilation should be avoided as much as possible due to the unwanted effects of increased PVR and decreased CO.[12]

SUMMARY

PAH is a lethal condition and the management of sepsis in patients with PAH is challenging. As the disease progresses, the right ventricle is susceptible to failure due to a high PVR. The limited ability of the right ventricle to increase CO in septic shock makes it difficult to deliver oxygen to the organ and tissues. Intravascular volume replacement and vasoactive drugs should only be considered after a thorough assessment. Priorities of care include improving CO and oxygen delivery by optimizing preload, reducing afterload, and improving contractility. Careful consideration must be given to administration of pulmonary vasodilators due to their potential to cause systemic hypotension. Lastly, mechanical ventilation should be avoided as long as possible because small changes in lung volumes can increase PVR and further decrease CO.

REFERENCES

1. Powers KA, Burchell PA. Sepsis alert: avoiding the shock. Nursing 2010;40(4):34–8.
2. Implementing the surviving sepsis campaign. Available at: http//www.survivingsepsis.org. Accessed November 16, 2015.
3. Chan C, Klinger JP. Sepsis and pulmonary arterial hypertension in the ICU. Adv Pulm Hypertens 2015;13(4):187–96.
4. Kurzyna M, Zytkowska J, Fijalkowska A, et al. Characteristics and prognosis of patients with decompensated right ventricular failure during the course of pulmonary hypertension. Kardiol Pol 2008;66(10):1033–9.
5. Vacca VM. On the alert for pulmonary arterial hypertension. Nursing 2009;39(12):36–40.
6. Hayes GB. Pulmonary hypertension a Client's survival guide. Silver Spring (MD): Pulmonary Hypertension Association; 2010.
7. Sztrymf B, Souza R, Bertoletti L, et al. Prognostic factors of acute heart failure in patients with pulmonary arterial hypertension. Eur Respir J 2010;35(6):1286–93.
8. Hoeper MM, Granton J. Intensive care unit management of patients with severe pulmonary hypertension and right heart failure. Am J Respir Crit Care Med 2011; 184:1114–24.
9. Cooper BE. Review and update on inotropes and vasopressors. AACN Adv Crit Care 2008;19(1):5–13.
10. Sole ML, Klein DG, Mosely MJ. Introduction to critical care nursing. St Louis (MO): Elsevier; 2013.
11. Urden LD, Stacy KM, Lough ME. Critical care nursing. St Louis (MO): Elsevier; 2014.
12. Zamanian RT, Haddad F, Doyle RL, et al. Management strategies for patients with pulmonary hypertension in the intensive care unit. Crit Care Med 2007;35(9):2037–50.
13. Kerbaul F, Rondelet B, Mott S, et al. Effects of norepinephrine and dobutamine on pressure load-induced right ventricular failure. Crit Care Med 2004;32(4):1035–40.
14. Hirsch LJ, Rooney MW, Wat SS, et al. Norepinephrine and phenylephrine effects on right ventricular function in experimental canine pulmonary embolism. Chest 1991;100(3):796–801.
15. Ducas J, Duval D, Dasilua H, et al. Treatment of canine pulmonary hypertension effects of norepinephrine and isoproterenol on pulmonary vascular pressure-flow characteristics. Circulation 1987;75(1):235–42.
16. Herget-Rosenthal S, Saner F, Chawla LS. Approach to hemodynamic shock and vasopressors. Clin J Am Soc Nephrol 2008;3:543–6.
17. Lier CV, Herban PT, Huss P, et al. Comparative systemic and regional hemodynamic effects of dopamine and dobutamine in patients with cardiomyopathic heart failure. Circulation 1978;58:466–75.
18. Pulmonary Hypertension Online University. 2015. Diagnosis and treatment. Available at: http//.www.phaonlineuniv.org. Accessed November 18, 2015.
19. Barst RJ, Channick R, Ivy D, et al. Clinical perspectives with long-term pulsed inhaled nitric oxide for the treatment of pulmonary arterial hypertension. Pulm Circ 2012;2(2):139–47.
20. Weisel RD, Vito L, Dennis RC, et al. Myocardial depression during sepsis. Am J Surg 1977;133(4):512–21.
21. Barnett C, Macheda RF. Sildenafil in the treatment of pulmonary hypertension. Vasc Health Risk Manag 2006;2(4):411–22.

22. Galie N, Hoeper MM, Humbert M, et al. Guidelines for the diagnosis and treatment of pulmonary hypertension: the task force for the diagnosis and treatment of pulmonary hypertension of the European Society of Cardiology (ESC) and the European Respiratory Society (ERS), endorsed by the International Society of Heart and Lung Transplantation (ISHLT). Eur Heart J 2009;30:2493–537.

Infection in the Critically Ill Older Adult

Jennifer Manning, DNS, APRN, CNS, CNE[a],*,
Jean E. Cefalu, PhD, APRN, AGNP-C, CWOCN, CFCN, CNE[b]

KEYWORDS

• Older adults • Infection • Critical care • Intensive care unit • Elderly • Sepsis

KEY POINTS

- There are many challenges in caring for older adults with infection in critical care environments.
- Older adults are at high risk due to diminished reserve, age-related changes, comorbidities, subtle clinical presentations, and institutionalization.
- Nursing care of the critically ill older adult with infection should be tailored to meet the unique needs of the critically ill older adult.

OVERVIEW

Infection is the invasion of a body or tissue by a microorganism. The infection may vary in severity and progress along a continuum. Incidence of infection increases with age in older adults, who account for 60% of the hospitalized cases.[1] There are many challenges in caring for older adults with infection in critical care environments due to increased risk. Older adults are at increased risk of infection due to age-related changes and associated infections.[2] The impact is increased mortality with 17% of older adult patients at risk for death compared with 2% of those older adults hospitalized for other problems. Older adults are at higher risk due to diminished reserve, age-related changes, comorbidities, subtle clinical presentations, and institutionalization.[3]

RISK FACTORS

Certain infections are important risk factors and may reduce quality of life. The infections, which present as a major risk for older adults, include pneumonia, influenza, tuberculosis, bacteremia, and nosocomial infections. Prevention strategies have been suggested in the literature, and improved implementation strategies are needed to play a major role in improving outcomes in older adult patients.[1]

[a] Nursing Department, School of Nursing, Louisiana State University Health Sciences Center, 1900 Gravier Street, Office 4B17, New Orleans, LA 70112, USA; [b] Nursing Department, School of Nursing, Louisiana State University Health Sciences Center, 1900 Gravier Street, Office 4A6, New Orleans, LA 70112, USA
* Corresponding author.
E-mail address: jmanni@lsuhsc.edu

Crit Care Nurs Clin N Am 29 (2017) 25–35
http://dx.doi.org/10.1016/j.cnc.2016.09.008
0899-5885/17/© 2016 Elsevier Inc. All rights reserved.

Pneumococcal

Pneumococcal disease is an infection caused by *Streptococcus pneumoniae*. Pneumococcal disease can result in pneumonia, sepsis, or meningitis and has been long recognized as an important risk factor in older adults. *S pneumoniae* bacteria are spread through direct contact, coughing, or sneezing.[3]

Pneumococcal pneumonia is the most common form of pneumococcal disease, accounting for 60% of the cases and 20% of nosocomial pneumonias. Pneumococcal bacteremia occurs in one-fourth of the cases of pneumococcal pneumonia. The older adult population experiences the highest pneumococcal rates of any population, wherein 50 per 100,000 are impacted. This rate is 3 times higher than the general adult population. The fiscal impact is significant because although the older adult requires hospitalization, the illnesses often result in complications. Sometimes other organ systems are impacted. The death rates from Pneumococcal bacteremia range from 0% to 80%. This percentage increases with age and patient comorbidities.[4]

Even though antibiotics are considered to be effective for treatment, death and complications often occur. Prevention methods, such as the pneumococcal polysaccharide vaccine and pneumococcal conjugate vaccine, can be effective as a cost-effective option. The pneumococcal vaccine is recommended for all older adults. The pneumococcal vaccine should be given after the age of 65 with revaccination after 5 years.[3]

Influenza

Influenza is caused by the *Haemophilus influenzae* bacteria strains. There are 3 types, A, B, and C. Types B and C are generally milder and do not cause pandemics. A is divided into subtypes and include H1N1 and H3N2. The influenza viruses change and create new strains, which can result in illness. Because of the constant mutation of the viruses, the annual vaccine must be regularly updated. Influenza A and B are major risk factors for older adults.[5] Epidemics occur each year, usually in winter. Health care costs are significant. Influenza leads all other illnesses in hospitals bed-days with older adults having the highest hospitalization and death rates from influenza of any population group. Eighty percent to 90% of deaths from influenza occur in the older adult population.[6]

Vaccines can provide protection against illness and are the best tool to fight influenza in the older adult population. Recent studies have reported the regular dose influenza vaccination reduced the risk of flu-related hospitalization by 76% in older adults.[6] The nasal spray vaccine is not approved for older adults because it contains live-attenuated virus.[7] Vaccine benefits are significant with substantial health benefits. The annual influenza vaccine is available each year starting in October and ending February. The trivalent inactivated virus standard or high-dose vaccine should be used. If the patient has an egg allergy, an allergist should be consulted before administering.

Nosocomial

Nosocomial infections represent any type of infection not present on admission to a hospital but develop after the third hospital day. Common nosocomial infections are caused by Staphylococcus, Pseudomonas, *Escherichia coli*, *Candida albicans*, hepatitis, or herpes zoster. The major types of nosocomial infections occur in the urinary tract, surgical wounds, blood, or lower respiratory infections, such as pneumonia. Other sites include nonsurgical wounds such as decubitus, intravenous sites, and the gastrointestinal (GI) tract. Incidence is greater in older adults than any other population group. Older adults have the highest rate of urinary tract infections, infected surgical wounds, and nosocomial pneumonia and bacteremia. Incidence rates for these infections increase each day of hospital admission.[8] There is a significant relationship between nosocomial infection in critically ill older adults and prolonged length of stay with the ultimate outcome of increased morbidity and mortality.[9] Rigorous infection control practices are needed in hospitals and long-term care facilities (LTCF).

Long-Term Care Facilities

According to the Centers for Disease Control and Prevention, approximately 1 to 3 million serious infections occur every year in LTCFs. Infections can range from urinary tract infections, diarrheal diseases, antibiotic-resistant staphylococcus infections, and many others. Approximately 380,000 patients die of the infections each year.[10]

It is not uncommon for intensive care units to receive critically ill older adults with infection from LTCFs. Critically ill older adults from LTCFs present as a unique challenge for intensive care units. This vulnerable population is associated with increased mortality, and for those overcoming the infection usually, this usually results in impaired long-term functional status.[11]

Strategies to prevent infection in LTCFs begin with prevention. Vaccination programs and strict infection control practice can help. In addition to influenza and pneumococcal vaccines, tuberculosis skin testing and booster immunizations should be implemented as needed. Other preventative measures include surveillance to identity infection control problems, monitor hygienic practices in food areas, regular monitoring of skin breakdown, aggressive treatment of skin breakdown, and minimizing use of catheters. Unfortunately, once a patient presents with an infection, such as methicillin-resistant *Staphylococcus aureus*, the course of treatment is challenging, complex, and often problematic.[11]

Other

In addition to the above-mentioned infection risk factors, other concomitant medical diseases are important to mention. Some of the most common chronic diseases include coronary artery disease, congestive heart failure, and chronic obstructive pulmonary disorders. In addition, older adults with malignancy or recent surgery are at increased risk for infection and a resultant critical care admission. Diagnosis of older adults is a challenge in various cases, such as tuberculosis, fever of unknown origin, infectious diarrhea, endocarditis, meningitis, and urosepsis and decubiti. Surveillance for infection in at-risk older adult clients is the primary strategy to improving outcomes. Unfortunately, because of age-related changes in the older adult and the concomitant conditions, older adults remain at high risk for the development of infection and subsequent admission to critical care units.

AGE-RELATED CHANGES IN IMMUNE FUNCTION

Immunosenescence refers to age-related physiologic changes in immune function.[12] The aging immune system is characterized by delayed and diminished responses to internal and external changes. The diminished effectiveness of the immune system places older adults at greater risk for the development of autoimmune diseases, cancer, and increased susceptibility to infection. The immune system is divided into 2 response systems, the innate or nonspecific immune response and the adaptive or antigen-specific immune response. The innate immune response includes first-line defense mechanisms, including the physical barrier of the skin, neutrophils, complement system, natural killer cells, and mucosal linings of the respiratory, GI, and urogenital tract. In older adults, even though the numbers of immune cells remain the same, the overall effectiveness is diminished, placing older adults at risk for a wide variety of infections, cancers, and autoimmune diseases.[13]

The adaptive immune response is more complex and relies on the recognition of an antigen and production of specific cells against a specific antigen. The adaptive immune system includes the T and B cells and cytokines. T cells differentiate in the thymus. Cytotoxic T cells contain CD8, which destroys pathogen-infected cells and cancer cells. Helper T cells contain CD4 that regulates both the cellular and the humoral immune systems and is important in reducing autoimmune diseases. Cytokines are proteins that serve as signaling mechanisms for the immune system. With advanced age, there is a general decrease immunity thought to be through the effects of reduced signaling by cytokines. The reduced strength of the immunologic response reduces the effectiveness of vaccinations, and the older adult may require multiple revaccinations to achieve immunity.[13] These changes leave the immune system unable to respond appropriately.

Respiratory System

Several age-related structural, physiologic, and immunologic respiratory changes put older adults at a distinct disadvantage over their younger counterparts. Bone demineralization secondary to osteoporosis precipitates some degree of vertebral collapse and kyphosis. Chest wall compliance is reduced because of calcification of the costal cartilages. The combination of kyphosis and reduced chest wall compliance gives the older adult a mechanical disadvantage to effective contraction and can impair the cough reflex.[14] The normal elasticity of the lung is replaced with fibrous tissue from environmental exposures to contaminants over time. Respiratory muscles decrease in mass and strength, and older adults become more prone to fatigue because of the increased work needed to breathe. Starting around age 50, elastic fibers around the alveolar ducts are replaced with fibrous tissue that results in the premature closing of the small airways, causing air trapping and hyperinflation, resulting in a gradual increase in the amount of anatomic dead space.[14] Pulmonary function tests normally show increased residual capacity, decreased vital capacity, and reduction in forced expiratory volume of approximately 5% to 10% per decade.[15]

The body's ability to regulate the respiratory rate to compensate for hypoxia or hypercapnia decreases with age. Hypoxia and hypercapnia often present with mental status changes often overlooked by clinicians.[15] During physical activity, decreased oxygenation combined with diminished ability to detect and respond to hypoxia results in decreased activity tolerance and delay recognition of respiratory disease or impending respiratory failure.[13] In addition, lung cilia decrease in number and activity, impairing the body's ability to clear secretions. These changes in the respiratory system of older adults often result in retention of secretions due to decreased cough and gag reflexes combined with diminished mucociliary transport, resulting in increased risk of aspiration, infection, and pneumonia.[14]

Endocrine System

Sex-specific differences related to infection risk are related to the endocrine system.[16] Men are much more susceptible to influenza and pneumonia and have an overall higher mortality than women.[17] Women, on the other hand, exhibit significantly longer life expectancies and have higher antibody response rates to vaccination.[18] Testosterone and estrogen exhibit significant effects on cells of both the adaptive and the innate immune systems. Estrogen tends to enhance immune system response, whereas testosterone suppresses the immune response.[16] However, after menopause, women lose the protective advantage, placing both sexes at increased susceptibility to infection.[16]

Changes in the endocrine system that impact susceptibility to infection are not necessarily normal changes with aging, but many older adults exhibit decreased insulin sensitivity and a delayed response to high blood sugar levels, which is exacerbated with critical illness.[19] Thyroid-stimulating hormone levels tend to increase but thyroxine and Triiodothyronine levels tend to remain at the low end of normal, accounting for slightly reduced metabolic rates and cholesterol metabolism.[19]

Nutrition and Gastrointestinal System

Sensory-motor function becomes slower with age throughout the body, including the GI tract. Some of these changes leave the older adult vulnerable to nutritional deficiencies and infection. Olfactory and gustatory function gradually decline, and up to half of older adults exhibit some degree of impaired smell and taste.[20] Tooth enamel becomes brittle, and the bone structure supporting the teeth loses density, causing tooth instability and breakage. Saliva is critical for maintaining oral health. Digestive enzymes in saliva inhibit bacterial overgrowth.[15] Although saliva production in healthy older adults remains constant, most medications taken by older adults have anticholinergic properties that reduce saliva production (xerostomia) and the condition is exacerbated when older adults take multiple medications. The loss of saliva promotes bacterial overgrowth, causing periodontal disease and pneumonia. Importantly, periodontal disease often extends systematically, and hematogenous seeding is the dominant cause of bacterial endocarditis.[21]

Peristaltic motion promotes continual clearance of food and pathogens through the GI tract. Increased tone and slowed peristalsis in the esophagus and stomach sometimes result in early satiety that reduces nutritional intake and can lead to malnutrition.[19] The pH environment and the natural flora of the GI tract inhibit bacterial growth. Reduced gastric acid production (hypochlorhydria) interferes with nutrient absorption and promotes bacterial overgrowth; however, reduction in gastric acid production is attributed to atrophic gastritis and *Helicobacter pylori* rather than normal age-related changes.[22] The gradual reduction in intestinal surface area changes the absorption rates of many nutrients (**Fig. 1**).

A gradual atrophy of mucosal surfaces along the small intestine coupled with a decrease in lymphatic follicles weakens immune function and increases the propensity for older adults to develop *Clostridium difficile* diarrhea.[22] Malnutrition contributes to overall decline in T-cell function. Protein calorie malnutrition is common in older adults especially during hospitalization and can lead to delayed healing and fluid shifts and increased infection.[22]

Changes in Immune Function

The thymus gland secretes thymosin, a hormone necessary for T-cell development and production. Lymphocytes pass through the thymus and are transformed into T cells during childhood. Once T cells mature in the thymus, they migrate to the lymph nodes. By age 75, the thymus is reduced to inactive fatty tissue. Involution of the thymus decreases the output of naive T cells, and antigen-experienced T cells accumulate but produce more proinflammatory cytokines, which contribute to a systemic proinflammatory environment in older adults.[16]

Neutrophils are the first immune cells to respond to infection, and although there appears to be minimal decrease in their abundance, their activity decreases with age. In younger individuals, neutrophils have a prolonged half-life at the site of infection, extending the phagocytic activity. However, in the older adult, the phagocytic activity

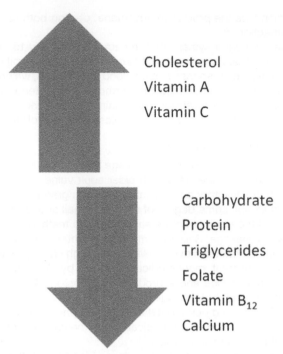

Cholesterol

Vitamin A

Vitamin C

Carbohydrate

Protein

Triglycerides

Folate

Vitamin B_{12}

Calcium

Fig. 1. Changes in nutrient absorption rate with reduction in intestinal surface area.

is reduced and neutrophils die prematurely.[19] Neutrophil effectiveness is inhibited by the release of cortisol. Cortisol is a glucocorticoid that elevates in the presence of physical and psychological stress. Acutely ill older adults are under extreme levels of physical and psychological stress, inhibiting an already weakened immune system.[13]

Integumentary System

The skin is a physical barrier that protects the older adult from infection. With age, the overall function of the skin slows. Epithelial cells produce enzymes and proteins that aid in phagocytosis of bacteria and inhibit microbial growth. Langerhans cells and melanocytes decrease in both number and effectiveness, increasing the occurrence of allergic reactions and sensitivity to sunlight. The epidermal/dermal junction flattens, decreasing overall tensile strength of the skin and placing the older adult at greater risk for skin tears and blister formation. The thinning of the dermal vascular bed contributes to the atrophy of the eccrine and apocrine glands. Reduced numbers of sweat and sebum–producing glands decrease the ability of the skin to retain moisture and inhibit bacterial and fungal growth. The subcutaneous tissue protects underlying tissues from trauma and aids in thermoregulation. The loss of subcutaneous tissue in malnourished older adults weakens the skin barrier and places the older adults at risk for pressure ulcers and infection.[15]

Cardiovascular System

The cardiovascular system undergoes several structural and functional changes related to age that reduce perfusion, thereby reducing the body's ability to respond to and fight infection. However, changes due to aging alone do not result in cardiac abnormality and do not affect daily activities. These changes present significant challenges during periods of stress (infection, trauma, surgery). In the presence of other risk factors (**Box 1**), the cardiovascular system becomes less efficient at maintaining homeostasis, and the process of delivering oxygen and nutrients to the tissues and removing and transporting waste is impaired. Structural changes include a decrease in number of cardiac myocytes with a concomitant increase in size resulting in increased thickness of the myocardium, especially the left ventricular wall. Sclerosis of heart valves impairs blood flow. Elastin fibers are replaced with collagen fibers, leading to ventricular stiffness and hypertension.[13]

Age-related changes in the electrophysiology of the heart are more prone to cause abnormality even in healthy older adults. These changes include a decrease in the number of pacemaker cells with an increase in irregularly shaped pacemaker cells in the sinoatrial and atrioventricular nodes and the bundle branches, thus increasing susceptibility to irregular heartbeats and arrhythmias, including atrial fibrillation.[19] Normal changes in an electrocardiogram in older adults include slightly increased PR, QRS, and QT intervals.[15] Diminished cardiovagal baroreflex sensitivity leads to blood pressure variability and an inability to respond to sudden changes in position or maintain blood pressure.[13] The resultant changes in perfusion of the heart inhibit the body's ability to adequately fight infection.

Genitourinary System

The bladder has several protective barriers against infection. Urine is usually sterile, and the high-osmolality, high-urea concentration, and low pH are protective against bacterial colonization. The regular flow of urine from the bladder is also protective because it decreases the time bacteria are in contact with the bladder epithelium and decreases the opportunity to attach and replicate.

In women, mucous production in the urethra serves to increase urethral resistance to leakage and prevent bacterial migration into the bladder. The periurethral and urethral areas contain beneficial flora, including lactobacilli, coagulase-negative staphylococcus, Corynebacterium, and streptococci that inhibit colonization of more pathogenic organisms. Menopause shifts the normal periurethral flora. Estrogen deficiency shifts the normal acidic vaginal pH to a more alkaline environment. Gram-positive flora is suppressed in an alkaline environment, and gram-negative bacteria proliferate. The loss of estrogen impacts the tissues of the proximal urethra and bladder neck, and they become thin and lose the mucous needed for coaptation. The combination of decreased mucous production and altered periurethral pH plays a significant role in the development of urinary tract infections in postmenopausal women.[15]

Box 1
Cardiac risk factors

- Hypertension
- Hyperlipidemia
- Inactivity
- Diet
- Smoking
- Stress
- Depression
- Obesity

In men, the prostate begins to enlarge around age 40; one-third of men experience symptoms by age 60, and half of all men exhibit moderate to severe symptoms by 75 years. The inability to completely empty the bladder increases urinary stasis, which places men at increased risk for complicated urinary tract infections as well as hydronephrosis.[15]

Age-related changes to the renal system include reduction in the size of the kidneys and renal blood flow but have little to no impact on renal function in the absence of acute or chronic illness. There is a gradual loss of nephrons, and the glomerular filtration rate is slowed in response to reduced perfusion.[19] Basal renin and aldosterone levels decline with age. A decline in the renal response to the renin-angiotensin-aldosterone system reduces the ability to respond to postural changes and correct sodium and potassium imbalances. Decreased sensitivity to antidiuretic hormone in the renal tubules impairs the older adult's ability to maintain fluid balance and leads to dehydration.[13]

NURSING CARE ASSESSMENT AND INTERVENTIONS

Nursing care and assessment should be tailored to meet the unique needs of the critically ill older adult. Older adults typically present with vague, atypical signs and symptoms. Some examples include nonspecific signs of infection, such as new mental status changes, increased falls, general malaise, anorexia, new urinary incontinence, nausea and vomiting, and mild tachypnea.[15]

Early recognition of symptoms is essential to ensure early interventions are aggressively pursued. **Table 1** depicts nursing care management and associated interventions strategies specific to the critically ill older adult with infection. Diagnostic evaluation should include chest radiography, echocardiography, and immune evaluation, as appropriate. Cultures should be collected for suspicion of infection.[13]

The cornerstone of aggressive treatment of critically ill older adults with infection is antibiotic therapy. In addition to antibiotic therapy, fluids should be provided to combat patient hypoperfusion as evidenced by hypotension, lactatemia, oliguria, and decreased oxygen saturation. Additional therapies should include the following:

- Vasopressors to treat hypotension.
- Corticosteroids, which can combat septic shock refractory to fluid resuscitation and vasopressor therapy.
- Sedation should be minimized.
- Ventilation when clinically appropriate based on respiratory assessment.
- Oral hygiene protocols should be implemented.
- Renal replacement for fluid and electrolyte disturbances.
- Glycemic control and enteral feedings.
- Deep vein thromboses prophylaxis.
- Stress ulcer prevention with low-molecular-weight heparin and proton pump inhibitors or H2 blockers.
- Careful monitoring for transition from sepsis to severe sepsis to septic shock.
- Respiratory: increase fluid intake to thin mucous sections.
- Deep breathing and coughing to aid movement and expand lungs.
- Oral hygiene to reduce microorganisms from invading the lungs.[8]

Removal of infectious sources should be continually evaluated, for example, catheters, implanted devices, abscesses, empyema, and surgical debridement. Early mobility protocols should be implemented. Patients should be positioned upright

Table 1	
Nursing care management and associated interventions for critically ill older adults with infection	
Management	**Intervention**
Early recognition	Monitor vague signs and symptoms

Diagnostic tests to identify infectious agent	Collect:
	    Complete blood count
	    Cultures (blood, urine, sputum, tissue, cerebrospinal fluid, as appropriate)

Imaging	Order:
	    Chest radiography
	    Computed tomography
	    Echocardiogram

Timely and appropriate antibiotics	Treat:
	    Gram-negative infections, which are most common
	    Monitor for increased multidrug-resistant pathogens
	    Ensure treatment within 1 h of suspecting infection

Eliminate infectious sources	Include the following interventions as appropriate: catheters, implanted devices, abscesses, empyema, surgical debridement
Early fluid resuscitation	Order: Crystalloids, fluid challenges
Vasopressor therapy	Treat: Persistent hypotension, hyperlactatemia, oliguria, decreased oxygenation
Immunosuppression	Order: Low-dose steroids
Supportive care for organ failure	Ventilation, renal replacement as appropriate
Prophylactic	Order: Low-molecular-weight heparin, proton pump inhibitors
Vaccinations upon recovery	Vaccines include influenza, pneumococcal (Greenberg,[4] 2016)
Limit catheter use	Urinary, vascular

when in bed to promote lung expansion. Vaccines should be evaluated for up-to-date immunizations. Patients should be ensured adequate rest and sleep in the critical care unit.

Nurses should implement standard precautions to minimize risk of exposure. As the older adult patient recovers, smoking cessation protocols should be implemented, as applicable. Strategies to promote regular exercise and a healthy diet should be provided.[8]

In addition to caring for the patient, nursing care should include caregivers and the family. Assessment and collection of information regarding onset and course of symptoms should be obtained. In addition, collection of the patient's history, past medications, and nonpharmacologic strategies should be documented in the patient's past medical history. The information collected from the family will assist with determining patient diagnosis as well as which strategies provide reorientation and comport for the patient.[23]

SUMMARY

In summary, critically ill older adult patients are at significant risk for increased morbidity, mortality, or long-term institutionalization. A disproportionate share of critical care resources used by older adults is projected to increase over the next decades. Many factors contribute to older adults increased risk, such as diminished physiologic reserve, aging process, comorbid illness, institutionalization, and decreased access to care. As part of the aging process, older adults often present with vague clinical presentation and atypical symptoms, which increase incidence of infection. The astute health care professional needs to be alerted that these vague symptoms may be an indicator of a more serious underlying illness trajectory.[24]

It is important to note that advanced age should not automatically preclude critical care admission, and older adult patients should be assessed similarly to patients in other age categories. Once an infection is identified, every effort should be made to provide aggressive care. In addition, determination of patient preferences (such as advanced directors, quality of life preferences) should be determined, and expectations about quality of life should be evaluated following discharge.[24]

REFERENCES

1. Dimopulos G, Koulenti D, Blot S, et al. Critically ill elderly adults with infection. J Am Geriatr Soc 2013;61(12):2065–71.
2. Manning J. Acquainting the critical care nurse with older adult physiological changes. Nurs Crit Care 2014;9(6):21–7.
3. National Foundation for Infectious Diseases (NFID). Facts about pneumococcal disease for adults. 2014. Available at: http://www.adultvaccination.org/vpd/pneumococcal/facts.html. Accessed May 1, 2016.
4. Greenberg S. Immunizations for older adults. 2016. Available at: https://consultgeri.org/try-this/general-assessment/issue-21. Accessed May 1, 2016.
5. Gravenstin, S., Mody, L. & Murasko, D. (2011). An interdisciplinary look at new developments in the prevention and treatment of influenza in older adults. The Gerontological Society of America. Available at: https://pogoe.org/sites/default/files/Pub%20Pract%20HD%20Influenza%20Final.pdf. Accessed June 1, 2016.
6. Talbot H, Zhu Y, Chen Q, et al. Effectiveness of influenza vaccine for preventing laboratory confirmed influenza hospitalizations in adults, 2011-2012 influenza season. Clin Infect Dis 2013;56(12):1774–7.
7. Centers for Disease Control and Prevention. Live attenuated influenza vaccine. 2016. Available at: http://www.cdc.gov/flu/about/qa/nasalspray.htm. Accessed April 30, 2016.
8. Funnel R, Koutoukidis G, Lawrence K. Tabbner's nursing care: theory and practice. 5th edition. Atlanta (GA): Elsevier.
9. Kaye K, Marchaim D, Chen T, et al. Effect of nosocomial bloodstream infections on mortality, length of stay and hospital costs in older adults. J Am Geriatr Soc 2014;62(2):306–11.
10. Centers for Disease Control and Prevention. Nursing homes and assisted living (long term care facilities LTCFs). 2016. Available at: http://www.cdc.gov/longtermcare/. Accessed May 1, 2016.
11. Mattison M, Rudolph J, Kiely D, et al. Nursing home patients in the intensive care unit: risk factors for mortality. Crit Care Med 2006;34(10):2583–7.
12. Ham RJ, Slolder Adultsne PD, Warshaw GA, et al. Ham's primary care geriatrics: a case-based approlder adultsch. 6th edition. Philadelphia: Elsevier Saunders; 2014.
13. Foreman MD, Milisen K, Fulmer TT. Critical care nursing of older adults: best practices. 3rd edition. New York: Springer Publishing; 2010.
14. Sharma G, Goodwin J. Effect of aging on respiratory system physiology and immunology. Clin Interv Aging 2006;1(3):253–60.

15. Miller CA. Nursing for wellness in older adults. 7th edition. Philadelphia: Wolters Kluwer; 2015.
16. Giefing-Kroll C, Berger P, Lepperdinger G, et al. How sex and age affect immune responses, susceptibility to infections, and response to vaccination. Aging Cell 2015;14:309–21.
17. Austad SN. Why women live longer than men: sex differences in longevity. Gend Med 2003;3(2):79–92.
18. Van Oyen H, Nusselder W, Jagger C, et al. Gender differences in healthy life years within the EU: an exploration of the "health-survival" paradox. Int J Public Health 2013;58(1):143–55.
19. Timiras PS, Navazio FM. Physiological basis of aging and geriatrics. 4th edition. New York: Informa, print; 2007.
20. Hummel T, Landis B, Huttenbrink KB. Smell and taste disorders. GMS Curr Top Otorhinolaryngol Head Neck Surg 2011;10:Doc04, ISSN 1865–1001.
21. Lopez J, Revilla A, Vilacosta I, et al. Valvular heart disease: age-dependent profile of left-sided infective endocarditis—a 3-center experience. Circulation 2010; 121:892–7.
22. Morley JC. The aging gut: physiology. Clin Geriatr Med 2007;23:757–67.
23. Cole M. Delirium in elderly patients. Am J Geriatr Psychiatry 2014;12(1):7–21.
24. Hartford Institute for Geriatric Nursing (HIGN). Abrupt change in mental status. 2016. Available at: https://consultgeri.org/patient-symptoms/abrupt-change-mental-status-0. Accessed April 11, 2016.

The Role of Liver Function in the Setting of Cirrhosis with Chronic Infection and Critical Illness

CrossMark

Susan Lee, MSN, APRN, FNP-BC*, Latanja Divens, DNP, APRN, FNP-BC,
Leanne H. Fowler, DNP, MBA, AGACNP-BC, CCRN, CNE

KEYWORDS

- Cirrhosis • Sepsis • Hepatitis C virus • Critical illness • Nursing • Nurse practitioner

KEY POINTS

- Chronic HCV-related cirrhosis places the patient in an immunocompromised state.
- Liver function normally plays a major role in immunocompetence and the clearance of toxins in critical illness.
- The patient with HCV-related cirrhosis and critical illness is at high risk for death in contrast to patients without chronic liver dysfunction.
- The patient with sepsis in the setting of HCV-related cirrhosis can have a more rapid decline in other organ dysfunction during critical illness.
- Registered nurses and advanced practice nurses can positively impact patient outcomes in the inpatient and outpatient settings in this population.

Without the insult of chronic organ dysfunction, the nature of systemic critical illnesses acutely injures multiple organs resulting in dysfunction. The patient with cirrhosis secondary to chronic hepatitis C virus (HCV), be it untreated or unresponsive to treatment, is at high risk for death and becomes more vulnerable to a higher severity of illness when critically ill. This article discusses the role of liver function in the patient with a systemic critical illness in contrast to the worsened pathophysiology of the patient with cirrhosis secondary to chronic HCV infection and critical illness, inpatient and posthospitalization management of the critically ill patient with chronic HCV-related cirrhosis, and the nursing implications and recommendations for future research for this population.

The authors have nothing to disclose.
School of Nursing, Louisiana State University Health Sciences Center, 1900 Gravier Street, New Orleans, LA 70112, USA
* Corresponding author.
E-mail address: Slee17@lsuhsc.edu

Crit Care Nurs Clin N Am 29 (2017) 37–50
http://dx.doi.org/10.1016/j.cnc.2016.09.006
0899-5885/17/© 2016 Elsevier Inc. All rights reserved.

BACKGROUND

Prevalence of Hepatitis C Virus Cirrhosis

Chronic HCV is the most common chronic, blood-borne infection nationally and is the leading cause of advanced liver diseases including cirrhosis, hepatocellular carcinoma (HCC), and liver failure requiring the need for liver transplantation in the United States. Approximately 184 million people are infected with HCV worldwide with an estimated 3.5 million people in the United States being chronically infected. There is an estimated 20,000 HCV cases resulting in death annually, which are often associated with cirrhosis or HCC. "In 2013, for the first time, deaths associated with HCV infection surpassed the total number of deaths from 60 other nationally notifiable infectious diseases."[1]

HCV is highly prevalent in specific populations including individuals born between the years of 1945 and 1965 ("baby boomers"); individuals who actively use or have a history of intravenous drug use; those who participate in high-risk behaviors (having multiple sex partners and unprotected intercourse); and socioeconomically disadvantaged and ethnic minorities including African Americans, Hispanics, and American Indian/Alaska natives. These aforementioned groups are considered to be vulnerable for reasons including a lack of access to care, inadequate disease management, a lack of awareness, and limited community and health resources. In addition to these factors, considering that HCV is silent in its course and progression, many cases are undiagnosed for years and thereby are untreated. When it is diagnosed, the cost of HCV treatment is often more than infected patients can afford leading to the decision to forego treatment and increasing their risk for the development of cirrhosis.[1]

Significance of Cirrhosis in the United States

Cirrhosis, an advanced stage of liver disease, is the 12th leading cause of mortality in the United States and is a common, comorbid condition of HCV. Cirrhosis results in fibrosis/liver scarring and nodular regeneration most commonly resulting from chronic liver injury sustained from chronic infection (hepatitis B or C), alcoholic fatty liver disease, and/or excessive alcohol consumption.[2] The condition complicates the management of patients with HCV infection and the condition leads to increased mortality.

There are two stages of cirrhosis: compensated and decompensated. Compensated cirrhosis is described as stage 4 liver fibrosis with or without the presence of esophageal varices; in compensated cirrhosis liver function is essentially preserved. Decompensated cirrhosis is defined as stage 4 liver fibrosis with the presence of one or several complications of portal hypertension including variceal bleeding, hepatic encephalopathy, ascites, spontaneous bacterial peritonitis (SBP), and/or hepatorenal syndrome.[3] Approximately 25% of individuals diagnosed with HCV infection in the United States have cirrhosis, which is often not diagnosed until there is an event resulting in decompensation.[1] Cirrhosis can significantly impact an individual's health status and quality of life predisposing the individual to multiple complications including HCC.

HCV infection and cirrhosis are commonly silent comorbid conditions. Individually these conditions have potentially severe complications associated with them. Together, these diseases increase the risk for severe complications with death being the greatest risk. The economic and patient/caregiver burdens of living with HCV-related cirrhosis are expected to significantly increase over the next 10 years despite advances in HCV treatment because of common barriers to treatment, such as a lack of access (high cost and a lack of insurance).[4]

Liver Physiology

The liver has many functions including metabolic processes, protein synthesis, and immune properties. Additionally, the liver has an important role in defending the body against stressful events and diseases during the inflammatory response. Such diseases as HCV result in chronic inflammation and the active production of acute-phase proteins (APP). APP are produced primarily in the liver in response to infection and inflammation and are regarded as important components of the innate immune response to infection. Hepatic APP have been identified as protective during times of an acute infection and promote the function of myeloid-derived suppressor cells, cells known for their anti-inflammatory properties in cancer. APP promote myeloid-derived suppressor cells mobilization, accumulation, and survival, and reverse dysregulated inflammation.[5,6]

In chronic HCV infection, chronic inflammation response facilitates cirrhosis progression. Chronic inflammation results in the normally smooth liver architecture being disrupted by fibrotic bands and disorganized nodules. It is known that the development of cirrhosis largely depends on two major factors: the patient's age and the patient's level of alcohol consumption. Additional contributing factors in cirrhosis development include oxidative stress, altered nuclear receptors, cytokine signaling, mitochondrial/peroxisome abnormality, hepatocyte apoptosis, and leptin resistance, which have been identified as mediators of progression toward inflammation and fibrosis/cirrhosis.[6] The chronic inflammatory response triggered by chronic infection therefore results in dysregulation and dysfunction. Further research is needed to identify the role of each contributing factor in the process particularly because cirrhosis is a reversible condition when the underlying condition is corrected.

Chronic Infection in the Setting Critical Illness

The patient with chronic liver disease becoming critically ill is at a high risk for death (**Table 1**). The pathophysiology of HCV cirrhosis places the patient at a disadvantage and without the capacity to defend against and withstand the insults systemic diseases place on the already immunocompromised host. Patients without cirrhotic liver disease have much lower critical illness mortality rates than those with cirrhosis.[7] Sepsis is estimated to be the leading cause of mortality and critical illness worldwide accounting for more than 20 billion dollars in health care costs.[8,9] The burden of disease that sepsis places on the patient without cirrhosis is high. When the patient with cirrhosis develops sepsis, the burden increases and care becomes even more complicated.

Table 1
Recommended vaccines for the adult with chronic liver disease, 2016

Vaccine	Dose 1	Dose 2	Dose 3
Hepatitis A	Day 1	6 mo	—
Hepatitis B	Day 1	90 d	6 mo
Hepatitis A/hepatitis B combo	Day 1	90 d	6 mo
Influenza	Annually	—	—
Pneumococcal vaccines PCV13	At diagnosis if never immunized up to age 64 y	—	—
PPSV23	65 y and older dose every 5 y	—	—

From Centers for Disease Control and Prevention (CDC). Vaccines that might be indicated for adults aged 19 years or older based on medical and other indications. United States. 2016. Available at: http://www.cdc.gov/vaccines/schedules/hcp/imz/adult-conditions.html. Accessed June 2, 2016.

Pathophysiology of Sepsis

Sepsis occurs when microorganisms, most often bacteria, are growing in the blood, releasing large amounts of endotoxin. Endotoxin is most often produced by gram-negative microbes and is a part of the structural make-up of the cell wall. It is released during the growth, lysis, or destruction of bacteria. It is important for the clinician to recognize that antibiotics stimulate the release of endotoxin and cannot prevent the toxic effects of them. Endotoxin release produces fever, induces the overproduction of proinflammatory cytokines, and is a potent activator of the complement and clotting systems.[10]

The dysregulated inflammatory response caused by endotoxins leads to hemodynamic alterations negatively impacting tissue perfusion to all organs. Global vasodilation occurs in an attempt to rush immunocompetent chemicals to the endotoxin resulting in a relative circulating volume loss and lower than baseline blood pressure. The lower blood pressure signals the neurohormonal response of increasing the heart rate to maintain tissue perfusion. Additionally, the endotoxin produced by the bacteria in the blood injures endothelial cells, the innermost layer of blood vessels responsible for facilitating blood flow, causing cell constriction, thus increased capillary permeability, and the release of nitrous oxide. Consequently, intravascular volume is then lost to the interstitial space via increased permeability and endogenous nitrate release perpetuates the vasodilatory state. Generalized third-spacing, or anasarca, and the hemodynamic changes mentioned previously lead to the hypermetabolic cellular state of apoptosis and lactic acid production most clinicians recognize as shock.[10]

New Definitions and Clinical Recognition Criteria for Sepsis

After much debate, the very complicated disease state of sepsis is now defined as "a life-threatening organ dysfunction due to a dysregulated host response to infection."[11] Urgent recognition remains vital to improving mortality rates; however, there is still no gold standard test for sepsis.[12] Before the new definition being developed, sepsis was thought to be recognized by systemic inflammatory response syndrome criteria (eg, tachycardia, tachypnea, pyrexia, leukocytosis, bandemia). Because such criteria were found to be nonspecific to the pathobiology of sepsis and not an indicator of the dysregulated response seen with sepsis, it became unreliable in the early recognition of sepsis. This means clinicians who once viewed sepsis as three phases (sepsis once recognized by systemic inflammatory response syndrome criteria, severe sepsis, and septic shock) must transform their thinking to recognizing sepsis using clinical criteria for organ dysfunction above baseline function. Fortunately, a valid scoring system is recommended to facilitate this recognition.[13]

The Sequential Organ Failure Assessment (SOFA) score grades abnormalities by organ system and accounts for clinical interventions (**Table 2**). A high score is associated with an increased likelihood of death. SOFA scores of 2 or more are associated with a 2- to 25-fold increased risk for death in comparison with patients with a score less than 2. Laboratory values are needed for full computation of this score and could delay early goal-directed therapy for those suspected to have sepsis. Therefore, the quick SOFA scoring system is recommended until pending diagnostics are available (see **Table 2**). The quick SOFA incorporates altered mental status and vital signs to identify patients who are suspected to have infection and are likely to have poor outcomes.[13]

Septic shock remains a subset of sepsis now being recognized by clinical manifestations profound enough to substantially increase mortality. These findings are persistent hypotension requiring vasopressor agents to maintain the mean arterial pressure

Table 2
Sequential (sepsis-related) organ failure assessment (SOFA) score

System	Score				
	0	1	2	3	4
Respiration					
Pao$_2$/Fio$_2$, mm Hg (kPa)	≥400 (53.3)	<400 (53.3)	<300 (40)	<200 (26.7) with respiratory support	<100 (13.3) with respiratory support
Coagulation					
Platelets, × 10^3/μL	≥150	<150	<100	<50	<20
Liver					
Bilirubin, mg/dL (μmol/L)	<1.2 (20)	1.2–1.9 (20–32)	2.0–5.9 (33–101)	6.0–11.9 (102–204)	>12.0 (204)
Cardiovascular	MAP ≥70 mm Hg	MAP <70 mm Hg	Dopamine <5 or dobutamine (any dose)[a]	Dopamine 5.1–15 or epinephrine ≤0.1 or norepinephrine ≤0.1[a]	Dopamine >15 or epinephrine >0.1 or norepinephrine >0.1[a]
Central nervous system					
Glasgow Coma Scale score[b]	15	13–14	10–12	6–9	<6
Renal					
Creatinine, mg/dL (μmol/L)	<1.2 (110)	1.2–1.9 (110–170)	2.0–3.4 (171–299)	3.5–4.9 (300–440)	>5.0 (440)
Urine output, mL/d	—	—	—	<500	<200

Abbreviations: Fio$_2$, fraction of inspired oxygen; MAP, mean arterial pressure.

[a] Catecholamine doses are given as μg/kg/min for at least 1 hour.

[b] Glasgow Coma Scale scores range from 3 to 15; higher score indicates better neurologic function.

Adapted from Vincent JL, Moreno R, Takala J, et al; Working Group on Sepsis-Related Problems of the European Society of Intensive Care Medicine. The SOFA (Sepsis-related Organ Failure Assessment) score to describe organ dysfunction/failure. Intensive Care Med 1996;22(7):708; with permission.

greater than 65 mm Hg; and having a serum lactate level greater than 2 mmol/L (or 18 mg/dL) despite adequate volume resuscitation. Hospital mortality is estimated higher than 40% for patients with these criteria.[13]

Chronic Liver Dysfunction in the Setting of Critical Illness

The liver normally plays a vital role in the systemic response to critical illness by the clearance of pathogenic organisms and toxins from circulation; and through acute-phase reaction (APP production) and release of liver-generated cytokines, inflammatory mediators, and coagulation cascade components. APP plays a significant role in reversing a dysregulated response to systemic inflammation. Some theorists suggest the normally increased circulation of bile acids and bilirubin may have a beneficial anti-oxidative or cytoprotective effect toward the fundamental aspects of energy and metabolic activity contributing to the stress response by inhibiting cortisol break-down.[14] Unfortunately, the degree of severity of liver dysfunction in the patient with cirrhosis decreases the likelihood of and capacity of the liver to function as it normally would in the setting of sepsis.

Gram-negative bacteria is the most common cause of sepsis in patients with chronic cirrhosis of all causes. Fungal coinfections are also common in this population because of their immunocompromised state.[7] Liver function in the setting of chronic liver disease and sepsis is associated with many prognostic factors. For instance, chronic liver disease impairs clearance of pathogens and medications administered thereby prolonging host exposure to disease and potentially toxic effects of medications. Impaired clearance of drugs can also compound or synergize pre-existing hepatic encephalopathy leading to the potential for oral intubation and mechanical ventilation for airway maintenance. Acute on chronic liver dysfunction also augments coagulopathy thereby increasing bleeding events with the potential for severe hemorrhage. Additionally sepsis, physiologic stress response, and hyperglycemia can facilitate cholestasis leading to an obstructive hepatobiliary pathology amid an already critically ill individual. Finally, acute on chronic liver dysfunction can convert the compensated patient with cirrhosis to a decompensated cirrhosis causing liver failure. Kidney failure secondary to sepsis in the setting of chronic cirrhosis potentiates liver failure and contributes to the prognostic indicators in this patient.

NURSING IMPLICATIONS
Role of the Registered Nurse

The critical care nurse must recognize the implications for the severity of illness in patients with a history of HCV cirrhosis in the setting of a critical illness, such as sepsis. These patients are at high risk for death and multiple complications during the intensive care unit stay. The critical care nurse must have prudent assessment and communication skills to adequately care for these patients.

Nursing assessment

The patient with cirrhosis is largely asymptomatic and often undiagnosed until decompensated and presenting to the hospital in multiorgan failure. These patients are most often admitted directly to critical care areas and can present with varying degrees of the common complications associated with liver dysfunction.

Using a head-to-toe approach, the nurse's assessments must be frequent and systematic giving consideration to the trend of findings. The nurse must consider the patient's risk for or actual state of hepatic encephalopathy by trending neurologic evaluations hourly. Frequent neurologic examinations are also necessary to detect findings associated with cerebral edema occurring secondary to increased capillary permeability and sodium imbalances.

Because of the potential for hemodynamic instability, interpretation and interval trending of vital signs must be monitored no longer than hourly. Adequate and early fluid resuscitation is an ongoing challenge compounded by the degree of severity of portal hypertension, hyperaldosteronism, and effects of sepsis in this patient. The nurse must anticipate this challenge to maintain adequate tissue perfusion.

In the setting of chronic liver disease and sepsis, the pulmonary system is vulnerable to an increased likelihood of noncardiogenic pulmonary edema. Manifestations of this condition on radiograph are characteristically described as a ground-glass appearance or diffuse patchy infiltrates. The nurse must recognize the significance of these results and connect this with the impact of the lungs' capacity to diffuse oxygen into the blood. The physiologic responses to chronic liver disease in the setting of sepsis (pulmonary edema, hemodynamic changes, and the inability to maintain a patent airway) are detrimental to the recovery of this patient and are responsible for worsened oxygen delivery, or tissue perfusion. Consequently, worsened organ dysfunction occurs in this patient more than the patient without chronic HCV cirrhosis.

In addition to the vital systems mentioned previously that must be monitored, the critical care nurse must also assess for ascites by measuring abdominal girth and trending it as needed, generalized edema, and strict intake and output measures. Output measures are often associated with accurate urine output measurement per urinary catheter. However, the nurse may also need to measure gastrointestinal output via gastric tubes or rectal tubes. In critical illness, a large amount of fluids can be excreted through the gastrointestinal tract. Ascites is another common finding in this patient that may be removed by paracentesis. The fluid removed must be calculated in the patient's output. Monitoring serial comprehensive metabolic panels also helps the nurse assess and trend hepatorenal function or compromise.[4]

Assessment of the gastrointestinal system can vary depending on the patient's presentation. The nurse must recognize the patient's likelihood of having esophageal or gastric varices secondary to portal hypertension even if the initial presentation did not include hematemesis. This patient is also likely to present with anorexia and/or dyspepsia. On physical examination of the abdomen with ascites, it is often round with striae on inspection. Auscultation of the abdomen may yield diminished to distant bowel sounds and percussion notes are often dull with a positive fluid wave. Deep palpation can be difficult secondary to the ascitic body habitus but may yield hepatomegaly and splenomegaly. Genitourinary findings are generally associated with dependent edema and gynecomastia in males.

Assessment of this patient's skin can present with jaundice (icteric), pruritus, spider angioma, and/or purpura or petechiae. Scleral icterus and nystagmus can also be seen on eye inspections. Jaundice in general is associated with poor prognosis and biliary obstruction. Pruritis is related to the stretching of the skin with edema or azotemia in the setting of renal function compromise. Spider angioma is sometimes benign but when multiple lesions are present, it is associated with liver disease and is attributed to the engorgement of superficial vessels. Purpura and petechial are associated with the thrombocytopenia accompanying advanced liver dysfunction and occur secondary to capillary rupture.

Nursing interventions

Endothelial injury occurring from endotoxin release in sepsis causes increased nitric oxide production and contributes to hypotension in the patient with sepsis. The crippling effects of sepsis in the patient with chronic cirrhosis exacerbates reduction of mitochondrial respiration leading to cellular death. Such factors intensify the deleterious effects of sepsis, thus increasing mortality for cirrhotic comorbidities.[15] As such, the critical care nurse plays an important role in titrating vasoactive pharmaceutical agents and volume support to increase cellular oxygen delivery and preserve viable organ function.

Because hepatic vasculature is already compromised, it is essential to maximize the oxygenated blood supply to the hepatocytes. Aside from monitoring laboratory studies to detect and track hepatic function, addressing nutritional needs is significant to support this hypermetabolic state. Enteral nutrition is identified in current sepsis guidelines as the best route for nutrition in the first 24 hours of care if possible. However, if the enteral route is not indicated in these patients, parenteral nutrition should be initiated within the first 48 to 72 hours.[16] Use of trickle feedings (infusing feeding no more than 10–20 mL per hour) via a gastrointestinal tube minimizes bacterial translocation from the intestine into the bloodstream. This strategy does not meet metabolic or nutrition demands but allows the accumulation of the gastrointestinal bacterial flora to be put to use and not further contribute to the patient's septic profile as an endogenous source of bacteria.[16,17]

Interventions should also include routine skin and wound assessment and care. Great importance is stressed regarding positioning and acknowledging the high risk for skin breakdown. Beds and devices providing pressure redistribution can assist in the prevention of nosocomial excoriation and pressure ulcerations. Patients who are hemodynamically unstable are at the greatest risk.

Nursing communication

Throughout the patient's course of illness communication and education remain important for the family unit. Often the underlying family processes are dysfunctional with regards to the patients' possible patterns of substance use and/or illness. The effects of the stress of hospitalization may further interfere with adequate coping mechanisms.

The nurse and/or social worker can intervene to help identify strengths, coordinate resources, and facilitate coping. Aside from establishing a unified family contact for decision processes, planning for discharge may include facilitating the unit with setting priorities and decisions with regard to the patient's coarse of hospitalization and care after discharge.

It is important for the nurse to provide information with regard to the pathophysiology and progression of cirrhosis. Ongoing follow-up and monitoring are necessary and lifestyle modification for the patient's best outcome. Topics should include when to prompt medical attention for ascites, encephalopathy, undue or spontaneous bleeding, and icteric presentations.

Finally, nursing communications to medical providers is also important. Bedside nurses remain with the patient 24/7 and often function as the medical provider's eyes and ears in their absence. Assessment trends and changes in condition must be recognized and communicated to the medical provider in a timely, succinctly, and objective way to modify the medical treatment plan appropriately in the patient's best interest. Nurses must also recognize when inappropriate medical orders are being given and clarify them with the provider accordingly, again, in the best interest of the patient.

Role of the Nurse Practitioner

The advanced practice nurse in the role of nurse practitioner (NP) must carry out the responsibilities of the registered nurse and a medical provider. The NP can play an integral role in disease management and health promotion in the inpatient and outpatient settings.

Inpatient management

Management of the critically ill patient with chronic cirrhosis and sepsis is complex and most often requires interprofessional efforts to ensure high-quality, safe, timely, and effective care. The NP must be credentialed to care for this patient in hospitals and skilled in the orchestration of specialist and staff collaboration on the case.

The critically ill patient with cirrhosis with sepsis most commonly presents to the critical care unit with multiple complications. Considering the acute and chronic aforementioned pathologies, this patient may decompensate more rapidly than those without the comorbidity of chronic cirrhosis. The NP must initiate and evaluate antimicrobial, pharmacologic, and intravenous fluid therapy closely to control the infectious source, stagnate the progression of the dysregulated inflammatory response, and facilitate oxygen delivery through hemodynamic support concomitantly.

Secondarily, the NP must be vigilant for the common complications associated with acute on chronic liver dysfunction, such as hyponatremia, encephalopathy, esophageal variceal bleeding, ascites, coagulopathy, and thrombocytopenia. Fluid resuscitation is necessary to replenish intravascular blood volume but also exacerbates extravascular fluid accumulation (eg, pulmonary edema, ascites, anasarca). Although increasing intravascular volume is necessary to maintain cardiac output and tissue perfusion, the pathology of this patient must be considered and the loss of intravascular volume into the third space recognized as ultimately counterproductive. Unfortunately, there is not enough evidence in the literature indicating the improvement of patient outcomes to support recommending the mobilization of third spaced fluids back into the vessel with albumin or other colloidal products.[16]

The role of the NP in the hospital setting can be as a hospitalist attending the case or as a staff provider on the critical care medicine service. Depending on the diagnostic and therapeutic procedures for which the NP is credentialed influences the specialty consultations required for the care of this population. For instance, a gastrointestinal specialist may be needed for variceal banding but not necessarily for paracentesis in the management and diagnosis of ascites. If the NP is functioning as the critical care/pulmonary provider, consultation for intubation and ventilator management are not necessary. Coagulopathies and thrombocytopenia's associated with this population usually do warrant the consultation of a hematology specialist to recommend safe treatment or replacement of factors or platelets. Sepsis guidelines also recommend infectious disease consultation for appropriate antibiotic stewardship. Otherwise, the management of hyponatremia, encephalopathy, sepsis, and shock fall well within the scope of the NP practice.

Outpatient management

Management of the patient with cirrhosis in the outpatient setting is critical to prevent any disease-related complications. In addition to monitoring liver and immunologic function, NPs are useful in improving symptom management, the prevention of disease-related complications, and in providing supportive care.[2] A large component of the care of the patient with cirrhosis and HCV is centered on prevention, specifically the prevention of further liver damage, systemic illnesses, and complications of decompensated cirrhosis.

Immunizations

It is essential for patients with HCV to be protected from any diseases that can weaken the immune system. The primary care NP assists in health promotion by ensuring all patients with HCV are up-to-date on all immunizations. Recommendations for vaccinations per specific guidelines from the Centers for Disease Control and Prevention in the chronic HCV population are noted in **Table 3.**[18]

System Management

Ascites

The natural sequela of cirrhosis includes the development of ascites, the accumulation of fluid in the abdominal cavity. Management of ascites is critical and includes diuretic therapy and a daily sodium restriction of 88 mmol or 2000 mg daily. Diuretic therapy with a potassium-sparing diuretic (spironolactone) with or without a loop diuretic (furosemide) is the mainstay of therapy. Compliance of diuretic therapy and sodium restriction is reinforced because ascites is associated with up to a 50%, 5-year mortality rate. Fluid restrictions are usually not necessary unless the sodium level is less than 125 mmol/L. Patients are also encouraged to refrain from alcohol consumption. A review of the current medication regimen is necessary to ensure potentially harmful

Table 3
HCV cirrhosis: symptom management

Symptom/Complication	Management Strategy
Ascites	• Daily sodium restriction, 2000 mg/88 mmol • Diuretic therapy: spironolactone with or without Lasix; initial dosage, spironolactone 100 mg with furosemide 40 mg daily, may titrate up to maximum daily dosages[2,19]
Infections	• Update vaccinations per CDC guidelines (see **Table 1**) • Thorough physical examination • Laboratory and diagnostics: CBC, blood cultures • Urinalysis with microscopy, urine culture • Chest radiograph, sputum culture • Pleural fluid culture • Ascitic fluid culture (all patients admitted to hospital with ascites) • Abdominal ultrasound[2,17]
SBP	• Complete physical examination • Laboratory and diagnostic studies (as stated previously) • Ascitic fluid culture • Empirical antibiotic (third-generation cephalosporin), usually when signs of infection (abdominal pain and fever) are present[2,17]
Hepatic encephalopathy	• Identify precipitating factors and correct cause • Lactulose 30 mL twice daily, with titration based on the goal of two to three stools daily • Add rifaxamin 550 mg twice daily to prevent recurrent hepatic encephalopathy[2,20]
Variceal bleeding	• Screening EGD shortly after diagnosis of cirrhosis • EGD yearly thereafter • Nonselective β-blockers for medium or large varicies • Uncontrolled variceal bleeding may require a postcaval shunt or TIPS • Prophylactic antibiotic: norofloxacin 400 mg po for 7 d (for recurrent gastrointestinal bleeding)[2,21]

Abbreviations: CBC, complete blood count; CDC, Centers for Disease Control and Prevention; EGD, esophagogastroduodenoscopy; TIPS, transjugular intrahepatic portosystemic shunt.
   Data from Refs.[2,17,19–21]

agents, such as angiotensin-converting enzymes, angiotensin receptor blockers, and nonsteroidal anti-inflammatory drugs, are either avoided or are used sparingly.[19]

Infections

Infections are a common complication of cirrhosis, occurring in approximately 25% to 30% of cases. Impaired immunity, immune defects, a high Child-Pugh score, variceal bleeding, low ascetic protein level, and a history of SBP are all risk factors for infection in the patient with cirrhosis and HCV. Because of the immunocompromised character of the disease, patients with cirrhosis are also 20% more likely to manifest a nosocomial infection. The most common infections in the population include SBP, urinary tract infections, pneumonia, endocarditis, and cellulitis.[17] These infections pose great risks including sepsis, multiorgan dysfunction, and death.

Management strategies regarding infections in the patient with cirrhosis and HCV are focused on prevention, early identification, and prompt treatment. The detection of SBP, a severe acute infection of the peritoneum that is highly prevalent and has a 30% to 50% mortality rate in this population, is extremely important. The NP must conduct a detailed physical examination that includes a general survey; vital signs; and a complete examination of the chest, abdomen, and skin. Laboratory and diagnostics are necessary and include blood counts and cultures, urine studies, chest radiographs, and an abdominal ultrasound.[10] Depending on the findings of the examination, additional diagnostic testing and/or procedures maybe warranted including an abdominal paracentesis. The primary care NP works closely with the hepatologist and interdisciplinary team to ensure that the risks of disease-related complications are minimized and treated promptly.[2,17]

Esophageal variceal bleeding

Recurrent variceal bleeding has a role in infection and is often a signifying event of disease progression. The mortality rate associated with recurrent variceal bleeding is 20% to 30%, 6 weeks post initial variceal bleeding. The incidence of a recurrent bleed is highest in the initial 2-week period after a bleed. Standard methods of care to reduce rebleeding are focused on the control of portal hypertension with the use of nonselective β-blockers and an esophagogastroduodenoscopy. If portal hypertension is not controlled and bleeding recurs variceal band ligation is needed. Recommended management for rebleeding after ligation includes surgical procedures for the placement of a postcaval shunt or a transjugular intrahepatic portosystemic shunt.[1,2] Bacterial infections particularly SBP increase the risk of early rebleeding It is therefore essential for the NP to initiate antibiotic prophylaxis to assist in reducing the incidence of bacterial infections, rebleeding, hospitalizations, and mortality. Norofloxacin, 400 mg twice a day for 7 days, is the first-line antibiotic therapy recommended for prophylaxis.[2,17]

Hepatic encephalopathy

Hepatic encephalopathy is a highly prevalent complication of cirrhosis that results in an altered mental status, neuropsychiatric impairment, and neuromuscular abnormalities. The condition is associated with substantial morbidity and mortality and is estimated to be present in 50% to 70% of patients with cirrhosis. The NP can assist in the identification, management, and treatment of the condition, which is targeted at reversing the episode. The American College of Gastroenterology recommends that the management of hepatic encephalopathy should focus on supportive care, and the identification and removal of acute precipitating factors, which might include infection, sepsis variceal bleeding, dehydration, constipation, dietary protein overload, and nonadherence to the lactulose therapy.[2,20]

Hepatocellular carcinoma

The NP must also initiate surveillance for HCC, the most common malignancy of the liver and the most common cause of death in patients with cirrhosis. HCC surveillance includes obtaining an abdominal imaging study (ultrasound, commuted tomography, or MRI) and an α-fetoprotein level every 6 to 12 months in the patient with cirrhosis. The interval for follow-up studies is based on the findings of the studies and disease-related risks.[2]

HEPATITIS C VIRUS TREATMENT AND CIRRHOSIS

Historically, HCV treatment in patients with cirrhosis, both compensated and decompensated, has resulted in poor treatment-related response, decreased tolerability, and low efficacy. The advent of new drugs, direct-acting antivirals (DAA), will potentially change the natural course of HCV, allowing eradication to be achievable in most patients. The presence and severity of cirrhosis does influence the likelihood of a sustained viral clearance. Patients with HCV cirrhosis, both compensated and decompensated, should be treated because the risk of disease progression, decompensation, HCC, and liver-related mortality are reduced. Every individual diagnosed with HCV cirrhosis should be referred and evaluated for treatment to improve overall patient outcomes.[21]

FUTURE RESEARCH

HCV cirrhosis has multiple associated risks including a reduced quality of life, the severe complications mentioned previously, and a high risk of mortality with decompensation or acute illnesses, such as sepsis. The new drug class, DAAs for HCV treatment, have been reported to aid in stopping the progression of cirrhosis. DAAs are being used to treat compensated and decompensated cases; however, treatment is not recommended for those with a short life expectancy that would not be improved by treatment.[22] Future research on the extent of cirrhosis after HCV treatment is warranted.

Another area for future research is fluid resuscitation in this population during critical illnesses, such as sepsis. Overresuscitation of intravascular volume is a common complication of sepsis in the patient without cirrhosis, but contributes to a more rapid demise of the patient with cirrhosis with sepsis.[8] The use of colloids specifically in the patient with cirrhosis with fluid volume overload should be studied for safety in the prevention of worsening associated conditions with sepsis, such as noncardiogenic pulmonary edema, anasarca, and ascites.

SUMMARY

The liver has many functions including metabolic processes, protein synthesis, and immune properties. Impaired liver function compromises the overall health of critically ill patients, but especially the patient with chronic HCV-related cirrhosis. Recognizing the liver's major role in immunocompetence, the toxic effects of inflammation and sepsis predispose the patient to complications and significantly increases their risk of mortality. Nursing has a critical role in the identification, treatment, and management of the patient with HCV and cirrhosis experiencing critical illnesses, such as sepsis. High-quality, timely, effective, and collaborative nursing management can improve the quality of life and the long-term outcomes for this population.

REFERENCES

1. Mera J, Vellozi C, Hariri S, et al. Identification and clinical management of persons with chronic hepatitis C virus infection—Cherokee Nation, 2012-2015. MMWR Morb Mortal Wkly Rep 2016;65(18):461–6.

2. Werner KT, Perez ST. Role of nurse practitioners in the management of cirrhotic patients. J Nurse Pract 2012;8(10):816–21.

3. Singh S, Fujii LL. Liver is associated with risk of decompensation, liver cancer and death in patients with chronic liver disease: a systematic review and meta-analysis. Clin Gastroenterol Hepatol 2013;11(12):1573–84.

4. Kanwal F, El-Serang H. Improving quality of care in patients with cirrhosis. Clin Liver Dis 2013;2(3):123–4.

5. Sander LE, Sackett SD. Hepatic acute phase proteins control innate immune responses during infection by promoting myeloid-derived suppressor cell function. J Exp Med 2010;207(7):1453–64.

6. Safaci A, Rezaei M, Arefi Oskouei A, et al. Protein-protein interaction network analysis of cirrhosis liver disease. Gastroenterol Hepatol 2016;9(2):114–23.

7. Galbois A, Aegerter P, Martel-Samb P, et al. Improved prognosis of septic shock in patient with cirrhosis: a multicenter study. Crit Care Med 2014;42(7):1666–75.

8. Vincent J-L, Marshall JC, Namendys-Silva SA, et al, ICON Investigators. Assessment of the worldwide burden of critical illness: the intensive care over nations (ICON) audit. Lancet Respir Med 2014;2(5):380–6.

9. Fleischmann C, Scherag A, Adhikari NK, et al, International Forum of Acute Care Trialists. Assessment of global incidence and mortality of hospital-treated sepsis: current estimates and limitations. Am J Respir Crit Care Med 2015;193(3):259–72.

10. Huether SE, McCance KL. Understanding pathophysiology. 6th edition. St Louis (MO): Elsevier; 2017.

11. Shankar-Hari M, Phillips GS, Levy ML, et al, Sepsis Definitions Task Force. Developing a new definition and assessing new clinical criteria for septic shock: for the third international consensus definitions for sepsis and septic shock (Sepsis-3). JAMA 2016;315(8):775–87.

12. Seymour CW, Vincent XL, Iwashyna TJ, et al. Assessment of clinical criteria for sepsis for the Third International Consensus definitions for sepsis and septic shock (Sepsis-3). JAMA 2016;315(8):762–74.

13. Singer M, Deutschman CS, Seymour CW, et al. The Third International Consensus Definitions for Sepsis and Septic Shock (Sepsis-3). JAMA 2016;315(8):801–10.

14. Bernal W. The liver in systemic disease: sepsis and critical illness. The American Association for the Study of Liver Diseases, 2016. Available at: www.wileyonlinelibrary.com. Accessed June 10, 2016.

15. Weigand J, Berg T. The etiology, diagnosis and prevention of liver cirrhosis. Dtsch Arztebl Int 2013;110(6).

16. Dellinger RP. Surviving sepsis campaign: international guidelines for management of severe sepsis and septic shock: 2012. Crit Care Med 2013;41(2):580–637.

17. Pleguezuelo M, Benitez JM, Jurado J, et al. Diagnosis management of bacterial infections in decompensated cirrhosis. World J Hepatol 2013;5(1):16–25.

18. Centers for Disease Control and Prevention (CDC). Vaccines that might be indicated for adults aged 19 years or older based on medical and other indications. United States. 2016. Available at: http://www.cdc.gov/vaccines/schedules/hcp/imz/adult-conditions.html. Accessed June 2, 2016.

19. Agency for Healthcare Research and Quality (AHRQ). Management in the adult patient with ascites due to cirrhosis. 2012. Available at: http://guideline.gov/content.aspx?id=45103. Accessed May 25, 2016.

20. Jawaro T, Yang A, Dixit D, et al. Management of hepatic encephalopathy: a primer. Ann Pharmacother 2016;30(7):369–77.

21. Garbuzenko DV. Current approaches to the management of patients with liver cirrhosis who have acute esophageal variceal bleeding. Curr Med Res Opin 2016;32(3):467–75.
22. Chen T, Terrault N. Treatment of chronic hepatitis C in patients with cirrhosis. Curr Opin Gastroenterol 2016;32(3):143–51.

Hospital-Acquired Infections
Current Trends and Prevention

Christine Boev, PhD, RN, CCRN, CNE*, Elizabeth Kiss, DNP, FNP-BC, RN

KEYWORDS

- Health care–associated infections • Hospital-acquired infections
- Ventilator-associated pneumonia • Surgical site infection
- Catheter-associated urinary tract infection
- Central-line–associated bloodstream infection

KEY POINTS

- Health care–associated infections (HAIs) are the primary cause of preventable death and disability among hospitalized patients.
- The Centers for Disease Control and Prevention monitors surgical site infections, central-line–associated bloodstream infection, catheter-associated urinary tract infections, and ventilator-associated pneumonias.
- Evidence-based prevention strategies are critical to decreasing HAIs.
- Nurses can work as a key member of the collaborative team to establish performance measures, test and study the initiatives, and work to decrease HAIs.

Health care–associated infections (HAIs) are the primary cause of preventable death and disability among hospitalized patients.[1] According to the Centers for Disease Control and Prevention (CDC), complications or infections secondary to either device implantation or surgery are referred to as HAIs. Specifically, the CDC monitors surgical site infections (SSIs), central-line–associated bloodstream infection (CLABSI), catheter-associated urinary tract infections (CAUTI), and ventilator-associated pneumonias (VAP). The purpose of this article was to explore HAIs specific to risk factors, epidemiology, and prevention, and how nurses can work together with other health care providers to decrease the incidence of these preventable complications. **Table 1** illustrates trends related to HAIs in intensive care units (ICUs). Mortality rates

The authors have nothing to disclose.
St. John Fisher College Wegmans School of Nursing, 3690 East Avenue, Rochester, NY 14618, USA
* Corresponding author.
E-mail address: cboev@sjfc.edu

Table 1
Health care–associated infections, incidence and prevalence

HAI	Mortality Rate, %	2014 SIR	2014 SIR Versus 2013 SIR, %
CLABSI	18	0.50	8
CAUTI	2.3	1.00	5
VAP	13	Not reported	Not reported
SSI (colon surgery)	3	0.98	5

Abbreviations: CAUTI, catheter-associated urinary tract infection; CLABSI, central-line–associated bloodstream infection; HAI, health care–associated infection; SIR, standardized infection ratio; SSI, surgical site infection; VAP, ventilator-associated pneumonia.
   Data from Refs.[1–3]

remain elevated for all HAIs with Standardized Infection Ratios (SIRs) increasing for CAUTI and SSIs, but decreasing for CLABSIs.

CENTRAL-LINE–ASSOCIATED BLOODSTREAM INFECTIONS

Reliable central venous access is necessary to manage and treat critically ill infants, adults, and children. On average in the United States, there are 15 million central venous catheter-days in the ICU alone.[4] There are 4 main types of central venous catheters (CVCs) that are used in the ICU. **Table 2** illustrates each catheter type.

Risk Factors

Several risk factors are associated with CLABSIs. See **Table 3** for intrinsic risk factors.

Extrinsic Risk Factors Associated with Increased Incidence of Central-Line–Associated Bloodstream Infections

- Increased length of stay before CVC insertion[5]
- Multiple CVCs
- Parenteral nutrition

Table 2
Types of central venous catheters

Catheter Type	Duration of Use	Insertion	CLABSI Risk
Nontunneled	Short-term use	Percutaneous insertion	Accounts for most CLABSIs
Tunneled CVC	Long-term use	Requires surgical insertion	Lower rate of CLABSI compared with nontunneled
Implantable ports	Long-term use	Requires surgical insertion and removal	Lowest risk of CLABSI
Peripherally inserted central catheters	Short to intermediate use	Inserted at bedside	Lower rate of infection than nontunneled CVCs

Abbreviations: CLABSI, central-line–associated bloodstream infection; CVC, central venous catheter.
   Data from The Joint Commission. Preventing central line-associated bloodstream infections: a global challenge, a global perspective. Oak Brook (IL): Joint Commission Resources; 2012. Available at: http://www.PreventingCLABSIs.pdf.

Table 3	
Intrinsic risk factors associated with CLABSIs	
Intrinsic Risk Factor	**Findings**
Patient age	CLABSI rates are higher among children and neonates compared with adults
Underlying diseases	Hematologic, oncologic, cardiovascular, and gastrointestinal diseases associated with higher incidence of CLABSI
Gender	Males associated with an increased risk of CLABSI

Abbreviation: CLABSI, central-line–associated bloodstream infection.
Data from The Joint Commission. Preventing central line-associated bloodstream infections: a global challenge, a global perspective. Oak Brook (IL): Joint Commission Resources; 2012. Available at: http://www.PreventingCLABSIs.pdf.

- Femoral or internal jugular access site
- Microbial colonization at insertion site
- Multilumen CVCs
- Noncompliance with maximal sterile barriers during insertion
- CVC insertion in an ICU or emergency department

Microorganisms can enter the bloodstream and contaminate CVCs through 2 mechanisms: extraluminally or intraluminally. The most common mechanism of entry is extraluminally, in which the patient's skin organisms at the insertion site migrate into the area surrounding the catheter tip.[6] Intraluminal contamination occurs from direct contamination of the catheter through the intravenous (IV) system (needleless systems, hubs, connections). Prolonged dwell time of the CVC is related to intraluminal contamination.[7] **Table 4** illustrates the microorganisms most commonly associated with CLABSIs.

Epidemiology

The CDC started collecting data on CLABSIs in the 1970s. CLABSI rates peaked in the 1990s and have steadily declined with state-mandated reporting of HAIs with the implementation of evidence-based interventions.[8] According to the CDC, CLABSI rates in the United States decreased 46% between 2008 and 2013.[1] In 2008, the Centers for Medicare and Medicaid Services (CMS) stopped reimbursing hospitals for costs associated with treating CLABSIs.[9] This change forced hospitals to look closely at evidence-based strategies to decrease CLABSIs.

Table 4	
Common microorganisms associated with CLABSI	
Microorganism	**Percentage of All Health Care–Associated Bloodstream Infections**
Coagulase-negative *Staphylococcus aureus*	31
S aureus	20
Enterococcus	9
Candida	9

Abbreviation: CLABSI, central-line–associated bloodstream infection.
Data from The Joint Commission. Preventing central line-associated bloodstream infections: a global challenge, a global perspective. Oak Brook (IL): Joint Commission Resources; 2012. Available at: http://www.PreventingCLABSIs.pdf.

The Agency for Healthcare Research and Quality developed toolkits to estimate both costs and mortality associated with CLABSIs. With an average mortality rate of 18% and a CLABSI rate of 5.3 per 1000 catheter-days, each year approximately 28,000 patients die of CLABSIs.[10] One estimate suggests that CLABSIs cost between $960 million and $18.2 billion annually.[11]

Prevention

Evidence-based prevention strategies are critical to decreasing CLABSI rates. Hand hygiene and aseptic technique are strategies known to decrease the risk of CLABSIs.[5,12] **Table 5** illustrates evidence-based strategies shown to decrease CLABSIs.

Each of the practices listed in **Table 4** are part of the Central Line Bundle developed by The Joint Commission on Healthcare Accreditation.[18] Consistent use of the Central Line Bundle has resulted in a 56% reduction in CLABSIs.[19] Other practices not included in the bundle that are associated with lower CLABSI rates include chlorhexidine-impregnated sponges[20] and alcohol-impregnated port protectors.[21]

Ventilator-Associated Pneumonia

Mechanical ventilation is a common treatment modality in the ICU used to treat respiratory failure secondary to a multitude of conditions. VAP is the most common complication of mechanical ventilation.[22] The incidence of VAP ranges from 2 to 16 episodes for 1000 ventilator days.[23] The most common organisms associated with VAP include *Staphylococcus aureus* (50%–80% of methicillin-resistant strains), *Pseudomonas aeruginosa*, and Enterobacteriaceae.[24]

Table 5
Evidence-based strategies that decrease CLABSI

Recommendation	Rationale
Catheter site selection: subclavian vein preferred	Upper extremity site related to decreased incidence of CLABSI compared with lower extremity[13]
Number of lumens	Use minimum number of lumens necessary[5]
Antimicrobial-impregnated catheters[14]	Recommended if comprehensive strategies to reduce CLABSIs is not working. These strategies include 1. Educating health care providers who insert CVCs 2. Use of maximal barrier precautions 3. Use 0.5% chlorhexidine for skin preparation before insertion
Maximal sterile barrier precautions	Includes sterile gown, sterile gloves, cap, and full-body drape[15,16]
2% chlorhexidine gluconate	Daily bathing with 2% chlorhexidine gluconate reduces CLABSI[17]
Advocate for catheter removal	Daily review of continued need for CVC should be done via multidisciplinary rounds; Zingg and colleagues[12] found that 4.8% of CVC days were unnecessary

Abbreviations: CLABSI, central-line–associated bloodstream infection; CVC, central venous catheter.
Data from The Joint Commission. CVC insertion bundles. Available at: http://www.joint commission.org/assets/1/6/clabsi_toolkit_tool_3-18_cvc_insertion_bundles.pdf. Accessed April 5, 2016.

From a financial perspective, the costs of VAP are tremendous. VAP is the second most costly HAI (second to CLABSI), adding an additional $40,144 per case.[24] More concerning is the estimated mortality of VAP, which is approximately 13%. This estimation is based on a meta-analysis of 6284 patients from 24 trials.[25] To decrease costs and save lives, the Institute for Healthcare Improvement (IHI) created a VAP bundle[26] that consists of specific evidence-based recommendations. These recommendations include the following:

- Elevation of the head of the bed between 30 and 45°
- Daily "sedative interruption" and daily assessment of readiness to extubate
- Peptic ulcer disease prophylaxis
- Deep venous thrombosis prophylaxis
- Daily oral care with chlorhexidine

Daily oral care is a new recommendation of the IHI bundle, and the evidence is conflicting. One meta-analysis of 12 randomized control trials (RCTs) revealed a 24% decrease in VAP rates with the use of 2% chlorhexidine.[27] This evidence is sufficient to support the adoption of this simple and relatively low cost option. Of recent interest is the effect of probiotics on VAP. One RCT with a sample of 146 patients noted a 47% decrease in VAP rates when daily probiotics were administered to ventilated patients.[28] Another intervention that has decreased VAP rates is the use of kinetic beds. Although costly, kinetic beds offer greater mobility of the patient and can also prone a patient with ease. One meta-analysis of 15 RCTs found a 53% decrease in VAP rates compared with traditional ICU beds.[29]

CATHETER-ASSOCIATED URINARY TRACT INFECTIONS
Costs/Mortality

CAUTI has been identified by CMS as a never event, and a condition for which hospitals no longer receive reimbursement for treatment.[30] There were approximately 93,300 urinary tract infections (UTIs) identified in acute care hospitals in 2011. UTIs are the fourth most common type of HAI.[1] Health care–associated urinary tract infections (HAUTIs) associated with indwelling urinary tract catheters account for 80% of UTIs.[30] CAUTIs account for more than 12% of hospital infections.[1] Between 15% and 25% of hospitalized patients may have an indwelling urinary catheter placed during their hospital stay.[31] The highest rates of CAUTI are identified in burn ICUs, followed by inpatient medical units and neurosurgical ICUs. The lowest rates are identified in medical/surgical ICUs. CAUTI can increase length of patients' stays, cost of patient care, and mortality. It is estimated that CAUTI contributes to more than 13,000 deaths each year with a mortality rate of 2.3%.[1] CAUTI accounts for 17% of hospital-acquired bacteremias, with an associated mortality of approximately 10%.[31]

Risk Factors

Indwelling urinary catheters are drainage tubes that insert into the urethra, sit in the urinary bladder and are connected to a closed collection system to drain urine. Indwelling urinary catheters are often a reservoir for multidrug-resistant bacteria and are often a source for transmission of infection to other patients.[31] The microorganism source can be endogenous from colonization of the meatus, vagina, or rectum. The microorganism source also can be exogenous from contaminated hands of the health care personnel, or contaminated equipment. The routes of transmission can be through the extraluminal route through migration along the outside of the urinary catheter, or by the intraluminal route through backflow of urine from a contaminated collection bag, breaks in the catheter-drainage tube junction, or biofilms of urinary microorganisms colonizing the urinary catheter.[31] In 1960, the closed sterile urinary drainage system was introduced into use. Even with a closed sterile system, breaks in the sterile system, urinary catheter biofilm contaminated with microorganisms, or extraluminal contamination can occur.[31]

The pathogens most often associated with CAUTI are *Escherichia coli* (21.4%), *Candida* (21.0%), *Enterococcus* (14.9%), *P aeruginosa* (10.0%), *Klebsiella pneumoniae* (7.7%), and *Enterobacter* (4.1%).[32] There are a substantial number CAUTI infections with multidrug-resistant organisms, which has made treatment of CAUTI difficult.

For a patient to be classified as having a CAUTI, the patient must meet all 3 of the following criteria, as outlined by the CDC.[1]

1. Patient had an indwelling urinary catheter that had been in place for more than 2 days on the date of event (day of device placement = day 1) AND was either:
   • Present for any portion of the calendar day on the date of event, OR
   • Removed the day before the date of event
2. Patient has at least 1 of the following signs or symptoms:
   • Fever (>38.0°C)
   • Suprapubic tenderness
   • Costovertebral angle pain or tenderness
   • Urinary urgency
   • Urinary frequency
   • Dysuria
3. Patient has a urine culture with no more than 2 species of organisms identified, at least 1 of which is a bacterium of ≥105 colony-forming units per milliliter. All elements of the UTI criteria must occur during the infection window period.

Prevention

Many indwelling urinary catheters are unnecessary. The risk for bacteriuria with catheterization is 3% to 10% daily, with almost 100% risk after 30 days of catheterization. It is estimated that 69% of CAUTIs can be prevented by following recommended infection control measures, which translates to 380,000 infections, and ultimately 9000 deaths each year prevented.[31] In 2010, through systematic reviews of 249 studies, Gould and colleagues[31] expanded on the CDC's current guidelines on prevention of CAUTI with the recommendations listed in **Table 6**.

SURGICAL SITE INFECTIONS
Costs/Mortality

Approximately 27 million surgical procedures are performed in the United States each year. SSIs account for 31% of all HAIs, making them the most prevalent HAI.[3] SSIs increase the patient's length of stay, interventions completed on the patient, readmission rates, the cost of health care, and ultimately place an increased burden on the patient.[3] The CDC's updated 2014 report on SSIs found a 17% decrease in abdominal hysterectomy SSI between 2008 and 2014, and a 2% decrease in colon surgery SSI between 2008 and 2014.[1] The additional cost of managing SSIs ranges from less than $400 for a superficial SSI, to more than $30,000 per patient for a deep organ/space SSI. SSIs were estimated to cost $20,785 annually and in 2009, the incidence of SSI was approximately 158,639.[33] SSIs have a mortality rate of 3%, with a 2 to 11 times higher risk of death directly related to the infection.[3] It is estimated that 40% to 60% of SSIs are preventable.[34]

Risk Factors

SSIs develop after surgery, in the location of the surgical site. The infection can be superficial when the skin is the only organ involved, or it can involve the tissue under the skin, organs surrounding the skin, or implanted material.[1] All surgical wounds have some degree of contamination that takes place at closure of the incision.[33] The pathogenesis of SSIs involves different factors, including the operating room environment, the host, the surgical procedure, and the specific microorganism involved.[3] Risk factors associated with SSIs include intraoperative blood transfusions, diabetes, and steroid use.[35] Bacteria are continually becoming more resistant to antibiotic treatment, making SSI prevention of utmost importance.[34]

Prevention

In 2002, the CDC and CMS collaborated and implemented the Surgical Infection Prevention Project to decrease morbidity and mortality associated with SSIs. What followed was a partnering of CMS, CDC, and other professional organizations nationally in what is known as the Surgical Care Improvement Project (SCIP). The SCIP highlights measurement of quality in 4 areas in which the incidence and cost of surgical complications is high, one of which is SSI.[36]

Evidence-based interventions to reduce SSIs were introduced through surgical care bundles.[33] The interventions include use of surgical attire, hand hygiene, antimicrobial sutures, preadmission showers and cleansing, and weight-based dosing.[33] In 2010, the Association of PeriOperative Registered Nurses (AORN) published recommendations for clinical practice to minimize risks for SSI, which included recommended practices for surgical attire. This brought about a surge of interest and research surrounding surgical attire in the operating room (OR), and the presence of personal items and food in the OR. The AORN recommendations are simple to incorporate into practice, and the Joint Commission uses these as expectations in their evaluations of hospital OR procedures.[33]

Hand hygiene of the anesthesiologists has been an area of needed improvement. Studies have linked anesthesiologists to direct transmission of pathogens to IV and anesthesia equipment. It has been recommended that all nonscrubbed OR personnel have access to alcohol-based hand rub.[33]

On closure of surgical incisions, it is unavoidable to introduce some bacteria into the surgical site. AORN has suggested the use of antimicrobial braided and monofilament sutures to reduce bacterial introduction into the surgical site. Daoud and colleagues[37] conducted a meta-analysis including 4800 surgical patients, which supported the reduction of incidence of SSI with the use of triclosan-coated sutures. In 2014, Singh and colleagues[38] created an economic model that reported that switching to triclosan-coated sutures had monetary benefits to hospitals, third-party payers, and patients, reporting a 10% reduction in SSI.

Preadmission showers with either 4% aqueous or 2% chlorhexidine gluconate (CHG)-impregnated polyester cloths kills 90% of skin staphylococci, including methicillin-resistant *Staphylococcus aureus* (MRSA).[39] Patient compliance with the preadmission showers, and standardization of directions for the preadmission showers has been an area identified for improvement. Edmiston and Spenser[33] developed suggestions for a protocol for standardization of preadmission showers, including electronic alerts for the preadmission showers that has improved patient compliance.

Another area for improvement includes weight-based dosing of preoperative prophylactic antibiotics. Current doses may be inadequate at inhibiting gram-positive

Table 6
CAUTI prevention recommendations

Who Should Receive Urinary Catheters	
When is urinary catheterization necessary?	Use urinary catheters in operative patients only as necessary, rather than routinely.
	Avoid use of urinary catheters in patients and nursing home residents for management of incontinence.
	Further research is needed on periodic (eg, nighttime) use of external catheters in incontinent patients or residents and the use of catheters to prevent skin breakdown.
	Further research is needed on the benefit of using a urethral stent as an alternative to an indwelling catheter in selected patients with bladder outlet obstruction.
	Consider alternatives to chronic indwelling catheters, such as intermittent catheterization, in spinal cord injury patients.
	Consider intermittent catheterization in children with myelomeningocele and neurogenic bladder to reduce the risk of urinary tract deterioration.
What are the risk factors for CAUTI?	Following aseptic insertion of the urinary catheter, maintain a closed drainage system.
	Insert catheters only for appropriate indications, and leave in place only as long as needed.
	Minimize urinary catheter use and duration of use in all patients, particularly those at higher risk for CAUTI, such as women, the elderly, and patients with impaired immunity.
	Ensure that only properly trained persons (eg, hospital personnel, family members, or patients themselves) who know the correct technique of aseptic catheter insertion and maintenance are given this responsibility.
	Maintain unobstructed urine flow.
What populations are at highest risk of mortality related to urinary catheters?	Minimize urinary catheter use and duration in all patients, particularly those who may be at higher risk for mortality due to catheterization, such as the elderly and patients with severe illness.
For those who may require urinary catheters, what are the best practices? Specifically, what are the risks and benefits associated with the following:	

Different approaches to catheterization?	Consider using external catheters as an alternative to indwelling urethral catheters in cooperative male patients without urinary retention or bladder outlet obstruction.
	Intermittent catheterization is preferable to indwelling urethral or suprapubic catheters in patients with bladder-emptying dysfunction.
	If intermittent catheterization is used, perform it at regular intervals to prevent bladder overdistension.
	For operative patients who have an indication for an indwelling catheter, remove the catheter as soon as possible postoperatively, preferably within 24 h, unless there are appropriate indications for continued use.
	Further research is needed on the risks and benefits of suprapubic catheters as an alternative to indwelling urethral catheters in selected patients requiring short-term or long-term catheterization, particularly with respect to complications related to catheter insertion or the catheter site.
	In the non-acute care setting, clean (ie, nonsterile) technique for intermittent catheterization is an acceptable and more practical alternative to sterile technique for patients requiring chronic intermittent catheterization.
Different catheters or collecting systems?	If the CAUTI rate is not decreasing after implementing a comprehensive strategy to reduce rates of CAUTI, consider using antimicrobial/antiseptic-impregnated catheters. The comprehensive strategy should include, at a minimum, the high-priority recommendations for urinary catheter use, aseptic insertion, and maintenance.
	Further research is needed on the effect of antimicrobial/antiseptic-impregnated catheters in reducing the risk of symptomatic UTI, their inclusion among the primary interventions, and the patient populations most likely to benefit from these catheters.
	Hydrophilic catheters might be preferable to standard catheters for patients requiring intermittent catheterization.
	Following aseptic insertion of the urinary catheter, maintain a closed drainage system.
	Complex urinary drainage systems (using mechanisms for reducing bacterial entry, such as antiseptic-release cartridges in the drain port) are not necessary for routine use.
	Urinary catheter systems with preconnected, sealed catheter-tubing junctions are suggested for use.
	Further research is needed to clarify the benefit of catheter valves in reducing the risk of CAUTI and other urinary complications.

(continued on next page)

Table 6
(continued)

Different catheter-management techniques?	Unless clinical indications exist (eg, in patients with bacteriuria on catheter removal post urologic surgery), do not use systemic antimicrobials routinely as prophylaxis for UTI in patients requiring either short-term or long-term catheterization.
	Further research is needed on the use of urinary antiseptics (eg, methenamine) to prevent UTI in patients requiring short-term catheterization.
	Further research is needed on the use of methenamine to prevent encrustation in patients requiring chronic indwelling catheters who are at high risk for obstruction.
	Unless obstruction is anticipated (eg, as might occur with bleeding after prostatic or bladder surgery), bladder irrigation is not recommended.
	Routine irrigation of the bladder with antimicrobials is not recommended.
	Routine instillation of antiseptic or antimicrobial solutions into urinary drainage bags is not recommended.
	Do not clean the periurethral area with antiseptics to prevent CAUTI while the catheter is in place. Routine hygiene (eg, cleansing of the meatal surface during daily bathing) is appropriate.
	Further research is needed on the use of antiseptic solutions vs sterile water or saline for periurethral cleaning before catheter insertion.
	Changing indwelling catheters or drainage bags at routine, fixed intervals is not recommended. Rather, catheters and drainage bags should be changed based on clinical indications, such as infection, obstruction, or when the closed system is compromised.
	Use a sterile, single-use packet of lubricant jelly for catheter insertion.
	Routine use of antiseptic lubricants is not necessary.
	Further research is needed on optimal cleaning and storage methods for catheters used for clean intermittent catheterization.
	Inset catheters only for appropriate indications, and leave in place only as long as needed.
	For operative patients who have an indication for an indwelling catheter, remove the catheter as soon as possible postoperatively, preferably within 24 h, unless there are appropriate indications for continued use.
	Consider using a portable ultrasound device to assess urine volume in patients undergoing intermittent catheterization to assess urine volume and reduce unnecessary catheter insertions.
	Further research is needed on the use of a portable ultrasound device to evaluate for obstruction in patients with indwelling catheters and low urine output.
	Further research is needed on the use of bacterial interference to prevent UTI in patients requiring chronic urinary catheterization.

| Different systems interventions (ie, quality improvement programs)? | Ensure that health care personnel and others who take care of catheters are given periodic in-service training stressing the correct techniques and procedures for urinary catheter insertion, maintenance, and removal.
Implement quality improvement programs or strategies to enhance appropriate use of indwelling catheters and to reduce the risk of CAUTI based on a facility risk assessment.
Examples of programs that have been demonstrated to be effective include the following:
1. A system of alerts or reminders to identify all patients with urinary catheters and assess the need for continued catheterization
2. Guidelines and protocols for nurse-directed removal of unnecessary urinary catheters
3. Education and performance feedback regarding appropriate use, hand hygiene, and catheter care
4. Guidelines and algorithms for appropriate perioperative catheter management, such as
  a. Procedure-specific guidelines for catheter placement and postoperative catheter removal
  b. Protocols for management of postoperative urinary retention, such as nurse-directed use of intermittent catheterization and use of ultrasound bladder scanners
Routine screening of catheterized patients for asymptomatic bacteriuria is not recommended.
Perform hand hygiene immediately before and after insertion or any manipulation of the catheter site or device.
Maintain unobstructed urine flow.
Further research is needed on the benefit of spatial separation of patients with urinary catheters to prevent transmission of pathogens colonizing urinary drainage systems.
When performing surveillance for CAUTI, consider providing regular (eg, quarterly) feedback of unit-specific CAUTI rates to nursing staff and other appropriate clinical care staff. |
| What are the best practices for preventing CAUTI associated with obstructed urinary catheters? | Further research is needed on the benefit of irrigating the catheter with acidifying solutions or use of oral urease inhibitors in long-term catheterized patients who have frequent catheter obstruction.
Silicone might be preferable to other materials to reduce the risk of encrustation in long-term catheterized patients who have frequent obstruction. |

Abbreviations: CAUTI, catheter-associated urinary tract infection; UTI, urinary tract infection.

From Gould CV, Umscheid CA, Agarwal RK, et al. Guideline for prevention of catheter associated urinary tract infections. Infect Control Hosp Epidemiol 2010;31:319–26; with permission.

and gram-negative bacteria associated with SSIs.[40] Historically, 1-g dosing of cefazo-lin prophylactically was standard protocol. Patients with a body mass index (BMI) of 30 kg/m^2 should receive a 3-g prophylactic dose of cefazolin 30 minutes before the first incision is made, and patients with a BMI of less than 30 kg/m^2 receive a 2-g dose of cefazolin 30 minutes before the first incision is made.[41] Currently not all hos-pitals in the United States have embraced weight-based dosing of prophylactic anti-biotics, which may leave patients vulnerable to SSIs. Further research is needed in this area, to prove efficacy of weight-based dosing.

Surgical attire, hand hygiene, antimicrobial sutures, preadmission showers and cleansing, and weight-based dosing are currently used to prevent SSIs. Other recom-mendations that have not been fully implemented as part of the SSI bundle include the following:

- Identification of patients who are nasal carriers of MRSA, and decolonization of these patients with mupirocin before surgery.[42]
- Irrigation of surgical wounds with 0.05% CHG.[43]
- AORN, The Society for Healthcare Epidemiology of America, and the National Institute for Health and Care Excellence recommend leaving hair at the surgical site and removing hair only if it is identified as interfering with the procedure.
  - If hair removal is necessary, it should be done outside of the surgical site, with single-use clipper heads, and hair should be cut, not shaved.[44]

Link to Nursing Care

Nurses are primarily responsible for ensuring that evidence-based interventions related to HAIs are implemented. Many of the HAIs are considered "nurse sensitive," meaning that the quality of nursing care is directly related to the incidence and prev-alence of HAIs. The nursing work environment is an important factor to consider when examining HAIs in critical care. Favorable nursing work environments are associated with fewer HAIs.[45,46]

HAIs are complex and multifaceted. It is crucial that the medical and nursing com-munity continue to investigate and implement evidence-based strategies to decrease the incidence and prevalence of HAIs both in the United States and around the globe.

REFERENCES

1. CDC. National and State Healthcare-Associated Infections progress report. 2016. Available at: http://www.cdc.gov/HAI/pdfs/progress-report/hai-progress-report. pdf. Accessed April 5, 2016.
2. O'Grady NP, Alexander M, Burns LA, et al. Guidelines for the prevention of intra-vascular catheter-related infections. Am J Infect Control 2011;39:S1–34.
3. Pedroso-Fernandez Y, Aguirre-Jaime A, Carrillo A, et al. Major article: prediction of surgical site infection after colorectal surgery. Am J Infect Control 2016;44:450–4.
4. Mermel LA. Prevention of intravascular catheter-related infections. Ann Intern Med 2000;132(39):391–402.
5. The Joint Commission. Preventing central line-associated bloodstream infections: a global challenge, a global perspective. Oak Brook (IL): Joint Commission Re-sources; 2012. Available at: http://www.PreventingCLABSIs.pdf. Accessed April 5, 2016.
6. Edgeworth J. Intravascular catheter infections. J Hosp Infect 2009;73(4):323–30.
7. Marscahll J, Mermel LA, Classen D, et al. Strategies to prevent central line-associated bloodstream infections in acute care hospitals. Infect Control Hosp Epidemiol 2008;29:S22–30.

8. Wise ME, Scott RD, Baggs JM, et al. National estimates of central line-associated bloodstream infection in critical care patients. Infect Control Hosp Epidemiol 2013;34(6):547–54.

9. Centers for Medicare & Medicaid Services. Eliminating serious, preventable, and costly medical errors-never events. 2006. Available at: http://www.cms.hhs.gov/apps/media/press/release.asp?counter=1863. Accessed April 5, 2016.

10. AHRQ. Tools for reducing central line-associated blood stream infections. 2015. Available at: http://www.ahrq.gov/professionals/education/curriculum-tools/clabsitools/index.html. Accessed April 5, 2016.

11. Unshield CA, Mitchell MD, Doshi JA, et al. Estimating the proportion of reasonably preventable hospital-acquired infections and associated mortality and costs. Infect Control Hosp Epidemiol 2011;32(2):101–14.

12. Zingg W, Imhof A, Maggiorini M, et al. Impact of a prevention strategy targeting hand hygiene and catheter care on the incidence of catheter-related bloodstream infections. Crit Care Med 2009;37(7):2167–73.

13. Merrer J, De Jonghe B, Golliot F, et al. Complications of femoral and subclavian venous catheterization in critically ill patients: a randomized control trial. JAMA 2001;286:700–7.

14. Rupp ME, Lisco SJ, Lipsett PA, et al. Effect of second-generation venous catheter impregnated with chlorhexidine and sliver sulfadiazine on central catheter-related infections: a randomized controlled trial. Ann Intern Med 2005;43:570–80.

15. Raad IL, Hohn DC, Gilbreath BJ, et al. Prevention of central venous catheter-related infections by using maximal sterile barrier precautions during insertion. Infect Control Hosp Epidemiol 1994;15:231–8.

16. Carrer S, Bocchi A, Bortolotti M, et al. Effect of different sterile barrier precautions and central venous catheter dressing on the skin colonization around the insertion site. Minerva Anestesiol 2005;71:197–206.

17. Shah HN, Schwartz JL, Cullen DL. Bathing with 2% chlorhexidine gluconate. Crit Care Nurs Q 2016;39:42–50.

18. The Joint Commission. CVC insertion bundles. Available at: http://www.jointcommission.org/assets/1/6/clabsi_toolkit_tool_3-18_cvc_insertion_bundles.pdf. Accessed April 5, 2016.

19. Marang-van de Mheen PJ, van Bodegom-Vos L. Meta-analysis of the central line bundle for preventing catheter-related infections: a case study in appraising the evidence in quality improvement. BMJ Qual Saf 2016;25:118–29.

20. Timsit JF, Schwebel C, Bouadma L, et al. Chlorhexidine-impregnated sponges and less frequent dressing changes for prevention of catheter-related infections in critically ill adults. A randomized controlled trial. JAMA 2009;301(2):1231–41.

21. Sweet MA, Cumpston A, Briggs F, et al. Impact of alcohol-impregnated port protectors and needleless neutral pressure connectors on central line-associated bloodstream infections and contamination of blood cultures in an inpatient oncology unit. Am J Infect Control 2012;40:931–4.

22. American Thoracic Society–Infectious Diseases Society of America. Guidelines for the management of adults with hospital-acquired, ventilator-associated, and healthcare-associated pneumonia. Am J Respir Crit Care Med 2005;171:388–416.

23. Barbier F, Adnremont A, Wolff M, et al. Hospital-acquired pneumonia and ventilator-associated pneumonia: recent advances in epidemiology and management. Curr Opin Pulm Med 2013;19(3):216–28.

24. Zimichman E, Henderson D, Tamier O, et al. Health-care associated infections. A meta-analysis of costs and financial impact on US healthcare system. JAMA 2013;173(22):2039–46.

25. Melsen WG, Rovers MM, Groenwold R, et al. Attributable mortality of ventilator-associated pneumonia: a meta-analysis of individual patient data from randomized prevention studies. Lancet 2013;13:665–71.

26. How-to guide: prevent ventilator-associated pneumonia. Cambridge (MA): Institute for Healthcare Improvement; 2012. Available at: www.ihi.org. Accessed April 5, 2016.

27. Labeau S, Van deVyver K, Brusselaers N, et al. Prevention of ventilator-associated pneumonia with oral antiseptics: a systematic review and meta-analysis. Lancet 2011;11:845–54.

28. Morrow LE, Kollef MH, Casale TB. Probiotic prophylaxis of ventilator-associated pneumonia. A blinded randomized control trial. Am J Respir Crit Care Med 2010;182:1058–64.

29. Delaney A, Gray H, Laupland L, et al. Kinetic bed therapy to prevent nosocomial pneumonia in mechanically ventilated patients: a systematic review and meta-analysis. Crit Care 2006;10(3):1–12.

30. Quinn P. Chasing zero: a nurse-driven process for catheter-associated urinary tract infection reduction in a community hospital. Nurs Econ 2015;33(6):320–5.

31. Gould CV, Umscheid CA, Agarwal RK, et al. Guideline for prevention of catheter associated urinary tract infections. Infect Control Hosp Epidemiol 2010;31:319–26.

32. Mitchell B, Ferguson J, Anderson M, et al. Length of stay and mortality associated with healthcare-associated urinary tract infections: a multi-state model. J Hosp Infect 2016;92(1):92–9.

33. Edmiston C, Spencer M. Patient care interventions to help reduce the risk of surgical site infections. AORN J 2014;100(6):590–602.

34. Spruce L, Spruce L. Featured article: back to basics: preventing surgical site infections. AORN J 2014;99:600–11.

35. Fukuda H. Patient-related risk factors for surgical site infection following 8 gastrointestinal surgery types. J Hosp Infect 2016;93(4):347–54.

36. Pham J, Ashton M, Kimata C, et al. Shock/sepsis/trauma/critical care: surgical site infection: comparing surgeon versus patient self-report. J Surg Res 2016;202:95–102.

37. Daoud F, Edmiston CE, Leaper D. Meta-analysis of prevention of surgical site infections following incision closure with triclosan-coated sutures: robustness of new evidence. Surg Infect 2014;15(3):165–81.

38. Singh A, Bartysch SM, Muder RR, et al. An economic model: value of antimicrobial-coated sutures to society, hospitals, and third-party payers in preventing abdominal surgical site infections. Infect Control Hosp Epidemiol 2014;35(8):1013–20.

39. Edmiston CE, Okoli O, Graham MB, et al. Evidence for using chlorhexidine gluconate preoperative cleansing to reduce the risk of surgical site infection. AORN J 2010;92(5):509–18.

40. Waisbren E, Rosen H, Bader AM, et al. Percent body fat and prediction of surgical site infection. J Am Coll Surg 2010;210(4):381–9.

41. Bratzler DW, Dellinger EP, Olsen KM, et al. Clinical practice guidelines for antimicrobial prophylaxis in surgery. Am J Health Syst Pharm 2013;70(3):195–283.

42. Perl TM, Cullen JJ, Wenzel RP, et al. Intranasal mupirocin to prevent postoperative Staphylococcus aureus infections. N Engl J Med 2002;346(24):1871–7.

43. Edmiston CE, Bruden B, Rucinski MC, et al. Reducing the risk of surgical site infections: does chlorhexidine gluconate provide a risk reduction benefit? Am J Infect Control 2013;41:549–55.
44. Burlingame B. Recommended practices for preoperative patient skin antisepsis. In: Perioperative standards and recommended practices. Denver (CO): AORN, Inc; 2014. p. e57–80.
45. Manojlovich M, Antonakos CL, Ronis DL. Intensive care units, communication between nurses and physicians, and patients' outcomes. Am J Crit Care 2009; 18(1):21–30.
46. Boev C, Xue Y, Ingersoll GL. Nursing job satisfaction, certification and healthcare-associated infections in critical care. Intensive Crit Care Nurs 2015;31(5):276–84.

Opportunistic Fungal Infections in Critical Care Units

Deborah D. Garbee, PhD, APRN, ACNS-BC[a],*,
Stephanie S. Pierce, PhD, RN, CNE[b],
Jennifer Manning, DNS, APRN, CNS, CNE[c]

KEYWORDS

- Invasive fungal infections • Critical care • Candida • Histoplasmosis • Aspergillus
- Cryptococcus • *Pneumocystis jirovecii* • Coccidioidomycosis

KEY POINTS

- Fungal infections are rare compared with bacterial infections, but they are on the increase in critical care units.
- Diagnosis can be difficult, resulting in increased mortality.
- Immunocompromised patients are at higher risk for fungal infections, including organ transplant, oncology, and human immunodeficiency virus/AIDS patients.

INTRODUCTION

Fungal infections have increased in the critical care setting.[1,2] Even though fungal infections are rare compared with bacterial infections, the mortality is higher.[3] Part of the rationale for an increased incidence of fungal infections may be an increased number of immunocompromised patients admitted to critical care.[1,2] Fungal infections are frequently referred to as opportunistic and/or invasive fungal infections. Opportunistic infections typically do not cause disease in persons with intact defense mechanisms.

The authors have nothing to disclose.
[a] Department of Adult Health Nursing, School of Nursing, Louisiana State University Health Sciences Center, Louisiana Center for Promotion of Optimal Health Outcomes: A JBI Center of Excellence, 1900 Gravier Street, 4A21, New Orleans, LA 70112, USA; [b] Department of Community Health Nursing, School of Nursing, Louisiana State University Health Sciences Center, Louisiana Center for Promotion of Optimal Health Outcomes: A JBI Center of Excellence, 1900 Gravier Street, 5A10, New Orleans, LA 70112, USA; [c] Nursing Department, School of Nursing, Louisiana State University Health Sciences Center, Louisiana Center for Promotion of Optimal Health Outcomes: A JBI Center of Excellence, 1900 Gravier Street, 4B17, New Orleans, LA 70112, USA
* Corresponding author.
E-mail address: dgarbe@lsuhsc.edu

Invasive fungal infections are diagnosed by deep tissue biopsy or sterile cultures.[4] Immunocompromised patients are at increased risk and include those with cancer, hematologic disease, organ transplants, and human immunodeficiency virus (HIV). Furthermore, sepsis patients sometimes become immunocompromised secondary to "...hyporesponsiveness, exhaustion, and apoptotic depletion of immune cells, increase in T-cells, and myeloid-derived suppressor cells".[5] Sepsis patients are frequently managed in critical care settings.

A review of literature was conducted on 6 fungal infections to determine incidence and prevalence, associated risk factors, best practices, and essential knowledge for critical care nurses. PubMed was searched using key words consisting of the 6 fungal infections: Candida, aspergillus, cryptococcus, histoplasmosis, P jirovecii, and coccidioidomycosis, fungal infection, and critical care unit. In addition, the Centers for Disease Control and Prevention (CDC) Web site was searched. Inclusion criteria were articles published between 2011 and 2016, involving adult patients, and the fungal infections of interest. **Table 1** reflects findings of the search.

INCIDENCE AND PREVALENCE

van Vught and colleagues[5] studied intensive care unit (ICU)-acquired infections in patients admitted with sepsis compared with ICU-acquired infections in nonsepsis admissions. They reported that, of 3640 admissions, 1719 were for sepsis and 232 (13.5%) were complicated by ICU-acquired infections.[5] Fungi accounted for 32 (9.6%) of these infections with the most frequently reported pathogens gram-positive (n = 151, 45.2%) and gram-negative bacteria (n = 89, 26.6%).[5] Infections developed more frequently in patients with higher Acute Physiology and Chronic Health Evaluation (APACHE) IV scores and Sequential Organ Failure Assessment scores.[5] Noninfectious ICU admissions totaled 1825 in the study period with 291 (15.1%) developing ICU-acquired infections; 22 (6.0%) were fungal infections.[5] Thus, even in the presence of sepsis, there were no significant differences reported in the 2 patient groups.

The CDC[6] reported that an estimated 46,000 cases of health care–associated invasive Candida occur yearly in America. However, the incidence varies by location and patient population; for example, 10 to 14 per 100,000 people are infected with Candida in Atlanta compared with Baltimore, respectively.[6] Furthermore, the CDCs Emerging Infection Program[6] identified Candida as the most common cause of bloodstream infections, which prompted the CDC to track this health care–associated infection (HAI). The goals of the Candida surveillance project are to

Table 1
Literature search results

Search Term	Results
Fungal infection and critical care units	141
Candida and critical care units	94
Aspergillus and critical care units	22
PJP and critical care units	9
Cryptococcus and critical care units	4
Histoplasmosis and critical care units	2
Coccidioidomycosis and critical care units	0

1. Track incidence of Candida and trends
2. Detect emergence and spread of resistance to antifungal agents
3. Determine the burden of antifungal-resistant Candida infections
4. Understand genetic mutations
5. Identify areas for prevention and interventions.[7]

According to the CDC,[6] *Candida auris* is an invasive infection that has emerged as a multidrug-resistant yeast and is associated with high mortalities in in-patient settings. It has been reported to cause wound and bloodstream infections as well as otitis, in patients of all ages. All of these factors can alter the natural defensive barriers for these patients favoring fungal colonization.[8] It was also noted that the age of the patient and various underlying diseases do contribute to patient vulnerability. Elderly patients with diabetes mellitus, renal insufficiency, and solid neoplasia have been associated with higher opportunistic infection rates.[4] Magill and colleagues[9] conducted a multistate point-prevalence study of HAIs at 183 US hospitals. A total of 452 HAIs were found in a sample of 11,282 patients. Of the total sample, critical care unit patients totaled 1707 or 15.1% and accounted for 156 (34.5%) of the total HAIs.[9] Candida was reported as the causative pathogen in 32 (6.3%) of the infections.[9] **Table 2** displays the 5 most common infection sites for Candida in the point-prevalence study.

According to the CDC, aspergillus[10] is not a reportable infection in the United States, and cryptococcus[11,12] is only reportable in a few states. Nonetheless, cryptococcal infection is the most prevalent fatal fungal disease worldwide, with sub-Saharan Africa having the highest incidence of 4000/100,000 in the HIV-positive population.[4] Cryptococcal meningitis is the most common disease in critical care settings. In critical care units, an incidence rate for invasive aspergillus has been reported as 6.1 to 57 per 1000 admissions.[4]

Histoplasmosis is more common in persons with HIV or AIDS particularly in areas where antiretroviral therapy is not readily available.[13] In Latin America, 30% of HIV/AIDS patients with a diagnosis of histoplasmosis die compared with estimated mortalities in the United States[13] of 4% to 8%.

The incidence of *P jirovecii* is estimated at 9% for hospitalized patients with HIV/AIDS and 1% for patients with organ transplant.[14] With treatment, the mortality is 5% to 40%, but without therapy,[14] the rate is near 100%. Schmiedel and Zimmerli[4] report an estimated 400,000 cases of *Pneumocystis jirovecii* pneumonia (PJP) each year. In a European study of HIV-positive and HIV-negative patients,[4] the incidence rate of invasive fungal infection with PJP was 1.5/100,000 with a mortality of 9.5%.

Coccidioidomycosis or valley fever had 8232 reported cases in 2014 down from an all-time high of 22,641 cases in 2011[15]; they accounted for an estimated 15% to 30% of community-acquired pneumonia in Arizona.[15] Mortality related to coccidioidomycosis in the United States between 1990 and 2008 averaged less than 200 per year.[15]

Table 2
Fungal infection in multistate point-prevalence study

Pathogen	Bloodstream Infections (n = 50)	Pneumonia (n = 110)	Surgical Site Infection (n = 110)	Gastrointestinal Infection (n = 86)	Urinary Tract Infection (n = 65)
Candida	11 (22%)	4 (3.6)	3 (2.7%)	3 (3.5%)	3 (4.6%)

Data from Magill SS, Edwards JR, Bamberg W, et al. Multistate point-prevalence survey of health care-associated infections. N Engl J Med 2014;370:1198–208.

RISK FACTORS

Numerous factors may contribute to patients acquiring opportunistic infections in critical care units. Many patients require the use of invasive tools; use of devices, such as humidifiers, have lines and tubes for monitoring, have disease processes that lead to decreased immune functions, and cross-contamination with hospital staff and other patients is possible.[6] Other risk factors for contracting Candida were discussed in consensus guidelines for treatment in ICUs.[3] The guidelines identified risk factors such as prolonged stay in ICU, Candida colonization, high APACHE II score, and blood transfusions. Very low CD4 counts, hyperglycemia, and corticosteroid and antibiotic use promote overgrowth of Candida.[8] It was estimated that, of patients in ICU for more than a week, one-half to two-thirds become colonized with Candida.[8] **Table 3** summarizes risk factors for each of the 6 fungal infections. Patients in critical care units have a higher risk in acquiring opportunistic infections due to conditions that require lengthy hospitals stays and invasive treatments. Patients having wound infections, peripheral or total parenteral nutrition, hemodialysis, catheter placement, prosthetic devices, or ventilators have a 5 to 10 times higher risk of acquiring an opportunistic infection than patients admitted in other areas of the hospital.[8]

Patient groups at risk for cryptococcus infection are immunocompromised patients, such as those with HIV, patients undergoing chemotherapy, or patients undergoing treatment for rheumatoid arthritis.[16]

People living in the southwestern United States, specifically California's San Joaquin Valley and southern Arizona, and parts of Mexico and South America, who may be African American or Filipino, are reported as more susceptible to coccidioidomycosis.[17]

Table 3 Risk factors for fungal infections	
Type of Fungal Infection	**Risk Factors**
Candida	Very low CD4 count Hyperglycemia Corticosteroids Antibiotics
Aspergillus	Chronic obstructive pulmonary disease Asthma, chronic bronchitis, or bronchiectasis Cystic fibrosis Hospital construction or renovation Contamination of air systems
Cryptococcus	HIV/AIDS Exposure to soil with bird droppings
Histoplasmosis	Immunocompromised patients by disease or treatment
P jirovecii	HIV/AIDS Chemotherapy patients Solid organ transplant recipients Rheumatologic disease
Coccidioidomycosis	Immunosuppressed patients Diabetic Pregnant California Central Valley prison population Living in San Joaquin Valley, southern Arizona, Mexico, and South America African American or Filipino decent

Data from Refs.[4,8,25]

In these locations, individuals who have additional risk factors, such as HIV/AIDS, are on immunosuppressive medications, have had organ transplantation, are diagnosed with diabetes mellitus, or are pregnant are at much greater risk at contracting coccidioidomycosis.[17] Coccidioidomycosis is found in dirt and dust particles, but once disturbed become airborne; therefore, people with occupations that are exposed to large amounts of dust are also vulnerable.[17] Coccidioidomycosis has also been found at increased rates in the California Central Valley prison population. Approximately 4000 California inmates were diagnosed with coccidioidomycosis since 2005.[18] **Table 3** reflects a summary of the common risk factors for invasive fungal infections.

OPPORTUNISTIC FUNGAL INFECTIONS
Candida

Candida is the most prevalent and common cause of nosocomial fungal infections in critical care areas.[19] Because of risk factors previously stated, patients in critical care are usually immunosuppressed, causing longer hospital stays, resulting in an increase in vulnerability to this fungal infection. Candida colonization is an overgrowth of the Candida on mucosa and skin. Candida has been associated with high mortalities and morbidities that account for 50% to 75% of cases of invasive fungal infections.[19] Early diagnosis has been shown to be key in having positive patient outcomes.

Clinical presentation
Candida species are normally found in the mouth, throat, vagina, and gastrointestinal tract. Weakening of the immune system by use of certain medications or disease processes cause Candida to multiply and cause symptoms of infection. Oropharyngeal candidiasis is known as thrush and presents when an overgrowth of yeast lives on the skin or mucous membranes. This overgrowth occurs when the inside of the mouth or throat becomes imbalanced and the yeasts begin to multiply. White patches or plaques are present on the tongue and other oral mucous membranes with symptoms of redness and soreness, difficulty swallowing, and cracking or sore formation at the corners of the mouth.[20] Vaginal Candida presents with burning, itching, and a "cottage cheese" like discharge. Imbalances occur when the normal acidity of the vagina changes and Candida multiply.[20]

According to Patolia and colleagues,[19] invasive Candida is the most common cause of bloodstream infections found in hospitalized patients. This infection results in long hospital stays, high medical costs, and poor outcomes. Inpatients are at higher risk for invasive Candida due to pre-existing medical conditions and present with chills and fever that do not improve after antibiotic treatment. This opportunistic infection can spread quickly to the heart, brain, eyes, bones, and joints if untreated.[19]

Diagnostic
Oropharyngeal candidiasis is diagnosed based on symptom presentation. Because Candida is normally found in the human mouth, cultures are usually not effective in supporting a diagnosis. Scrapings are taken from the infected areas and examined under a microscope for overgrowth. Vaginal candidiasis is diagnosed by taking samples of vaginal secretions and examining for yeast count under a microscope. In invasive candidiasis, a blood culture is used to confirm the diagnosis.[21]

Aspergillus

Aspergillus is a fungal infection that usually presents in immunocompromised hosts. This fungal infection can often present as invasive aspergillosis (IA) in critically ill patients. Although rare in occurrence, patients with IA experience a higher mortality[22] of up to 60% to 90%.

Clinical presentation

There are no specific clinical symptoms for IA in at-risk groups. Early signs of infection include fever or cough. Hemoptysis may or may not be present. Clinicians should be alerted early in high-risk patients if pulmonary symptoms are noted because this may indicate pulmonary infarction due to lung infection with IA.[4] Typically, patients present with deteriorating conditions. Later clinical signs include seizures or alteration in neurologic function. Manifestations in extrapulmonary organs are rare.[4]

Diagnostic

The gold standard for diagnosis is a culture. Obtaining culture results is a challenge because of the time it takes to obtain results, typically, as long as days to weeks. Polymerase chain reaction (PCR) may be a useful alternative in diagnoses because this diagnostic test has high levels of sensitivity and specificity.[4] Diagnostic imaging is typically used to support early evidence of IA. When nodules or lesions are noted in the imaging results, the clinician should be alerted to further assess the patient to ensure timely treatment is provided.[4]

Cryptococcus

Cryptococcus is an encapsulated yeast located in the ground, mostly in soil. When a person inhales cryptococcus spores, there are usually no symptoms. Cryptococcal disease often manifests when a latent infection reactivates when the person becomes immunosuppressed. The most common manifestations are meningitis and pneumonia.[23]

Clinical presentation

Similar to the other fungal infections, there are no specific symptoms for cryptococcus fungal infection. Because early treatment is desirable, a variety of clinical features could signal the clinician to the possibility of a fungal infection. Other than presenting with general infection symptoms, patients will typically present with symptoms in the respiratory or neurologic systems. General symptoms include slow resolution of infection to common treatments, mild to moderate fever, malaise, cough, and pleuritic pain.[2] The patient may report a nonproductive or productive cough. In rare instances, the patient may present with hemoptysis, rales, plural rub, or plural effusions.[2] Without prompt treatment, the patient may develop respiratory distress syndrome.

In the neurologic system, meningitis symptoms are the most common manifestation. These symptoms include headache and altered mental status. Other vague symptoms include personality changes, confusion, lethargy, obtundation, and coma.[2] Nausea and vomiting are common as well as fever and reports of a "stiff neck."[2] If the clinician is not astute to prompt treatment, this type of infection will often be fatal within weeks of onset. In severely immunocompromised patients, fever may not be present or may be very mild. Some patients may report blurred vision, diplopia, and photophobia as well as hearing defects, seizures, ataxia, and aphasia.[2] Hydrocephalus is a late complication.[2]

In addition to respiratory and neurologic symptoms, other signs of infection may be noted in the skin, prostate, and bones.[2] The presenting manifestations include papules, pustules, nodules, ulcers, or draining sinuses.[2] In post–organ transplant patients, cellulitis with necrotizing vasculitis may be noted in the clinical presentation. In the bone, presentations may include abscesses. Typically, patients are severely immunocompromised with profound neutropenia, low CD4 counts in poorly controlled HIV patients, and receiving corticosteroids and/or chemotherapy.[2] Other at-risk patients include those with chronic renal and liver disease, poorly controlled diabetics, or lung disease, such as chronic obstructive pulmonary disease, bronchiectasis, and cystic fibrosis.[2] One must also consider the area of residence and recent travel of the client.

Diagnostic

Cryptococcus is difficult to diagnose, and early treatment is key to improved patient outcomes. Most diagnostic tests are nonspecific, and cultures take time to complete. Early suspicion of a fungal infection should be followed with antifungal therapy to ensure positive outcomes for the patient and prevent further development of an invasive fungal infection. The mortality for patients who develop invasive fungal infections such as cryptococcus is high. There is no rapid diagnostic test for Cryptococcus.[24] Cultures may require days to weeks to identify an organism.[2]

Histoplasmosis

Histoplasmosis is endemic to river valleys of the Ohio, Missouri, Mississippi, and some Central American river valleys.[2] Histoplasmosis is also known as Darling disease and is found in soil inhabited by bats and birds.[25] The respiratory tract is the portal of entry. A patient with a healthy immune system can control the infection. However, histoplasmosis can spread via the lymphatics to areas such as the liver, spleen, bone marrow, adrenals, and gastrointestinal system.[25]

Clinical presentation

Pulmonary nodules, broncholithiasis, fibrosing mediastinitis, or pneumonia may be presenting symptoms.[2] Fibrosing mediastinitis is not common, but can be fatal.[2] In asymptomatic patients, malignancy must be ruled out.

Diagnostic

In the case of pulmonary histoplasmosis infections, diagnostic tests may include blood tests for antigens and PCRs; radiographic tests such as computed tomography and PET; and invasive procedures for biopsies include bronchoscopy, mediastinoscopy, and/or video-assisted thorascopy.[2]

Pneumocystis jirovecii

P jirovecii was formerly referred to as *Pneumocystis carinii*.[25] It was originally identified as a protozoan, but is now proven to belong to the fungi family.[4] It is often seen in AIDS patients and other immunocompromised patients. *P jirovecii* is normally present in the respiratory tract, but proliferates in the lungs of immunocompromised patients.[25]

Clinical presentation

Immunocompromised patients are susceptible to *P jirovecii*.[2] HIV-positive patients have a prolonged onset of PJP, whereas non-HIV patient's onset is more severe and sudden, with a higher mortality.[4] The cascade of symptoms[1,4] is displayed in **Fig. 1**. These symptoms can progress to pneumothorax. Onset of infection with PJP should prompt the health care provider to search the cause, such as HIV infection, malignancy, cytotoxic agents, or immune suppressants.[2]

In immunosuppressed patients, PJP is the most prevalent opportunistic infection.[7] Kim and colleagues[26] sought to discover prognostic factors for PJP in HIV-negative patients. Clinical presentation includes fever, cough, sputum, and dyspnea. The investigators studied 173 non-HIV-positive patients with PJP and reported that high alveolar-arterial oxygen gradient, bacteremia, increased blood urea nitrogen (BUN),

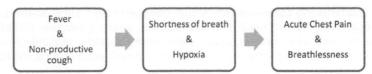

Fig. 1. Cascade of symptoms for PJP. (*Data from* Bajwa SJ, Kulshrestha A. Fungal infections in intensive care unit: challenges in diagnosis and management. Ann Med Health Sci Res 2013;3:238–44; and Schmiedel Y, Zimmerli S. Common invasive fungal diseases: an overview of invasive candidiasis, aspergillosis, cryptococcosis, and pneumocystis pneumonia. Swiss Med Wkly 2016;146:w14281.)

and pre-existing lung disease were indicators of poor prognosis.[26] In a retrospective study, Li and colleagues[27] reported that PJP in non-HIV patients were associated with delay in antimicrobial therapy and poor prognosis.

Diagnostic
Diagnosis of PJP is made based on clinical symptoms, positive direct fluorescent antibody, and PCR from sputum or bronchoalveolar lavage fluid.[4] Chest radiography or computed tomography may reveal bilateral ground glass opacity[4,26] or pulmonary infiltrates.[1,4] Serum $(1–3)$-β-D-glucan is a marker with a 96% sensitivity and 87% specificity that can be useful for diagnosis in patients that cannot undergo bronchoscopy.[4]

Coccidioidomycosis

Coccidioidomycosis (cocci) or valley fever is caused by inhaling fungal spores into the lungs, which then lodges in the air sacs. The spores reproduce, and mini spores are formed. These mini spores then burst, releasing hundreds of new spores. The tissue becomes inflamed as the fungus continues this reproductive cycle.[18] Ferry[18] estimated that cocci infections have killed more Americans than West Nile virus, rabies, and Ebola combined. Approximately 20,000 Americans contract coccidioidomycosis annually, contributing to an underestimated average of 170 deaths. The incidence of this fungal infection has risen from 2271 reported cases in 1998 to 22,641 reported cases in 2011.[18] Contributing to this increase has been the ideal climate for cultivating cocci spores: burst of rain followed by long dry spells, which result in the soil remaining arid and parched. Southern California winds then pick up the spore-filled dust and transmit cocci spores with ease.[18]

Clinical presentation
According to the CDC,[17] coccidioidomycosis is a fungal infection usually found in the lungs, but can spread quickly to other parts of the body. Coccidioidomycosis is an infection caused by breathing in microscopic fungal spores found in the air from dust particles in the southwestern United States, parts of Mexico, and Central and South America. Patients exposed to high dust and after earthquakes in these geographic areas are at increased risk. Usually 1 to 3 weeks after exposure, patients will present with fever, fatigue, cough, dyspnea, headache, night sweats, muscle pain, loss of consciousness, weakness, and a rash.[17]

Diagnostic
Blood testing is the most common diagnostic tool. Serology testing is done to detect immunoglobulin M (IgM) and IgG antibodies in patients suspected of coccidioidomycosis. Other testing includes testing for enzyme immunoassay, immunodiffusion, complement fixation, a respiratory tissue culture, using a microscope to detect

spherules in tissue, and urinary antigen detection in the most severe cases with immunocompromised patients.[21]

TREATMENT

As with any infection, treatment is based on the causative organism and severity of the disease. Two main antifungal classes exist along with novel agents. Polyenes and triazoles are the major classes and novel agents include echinocandins and extended-spectrum triazoles.[2] **Table 4** presents information on drug classifications, and **Table 5** shows treatment comparisons.

Candida Management

Determining the specific species of Candida is essential to guide in the development of the right antifungal treatment. Fluconazole is good for treatment of Candida albicans.[2] Posaconazole is used for prophylaxis against invasive fungal infections of oropharyngeal Candida.[2,4] Severe cases of Candida or those that are azole-resistant are treated with amphotericin B. Vaginal Candida is usually treated with antifungal vaginal suppositories or creams. The length of the treatment with creams and suppositories can range from 1 to 7 days. Mild or moderate infections can be treated with a single dose of oral antifungal medication. These types of medications usually work in 80% to 90% of Candida cases; however, some resistant infections require a lengthier treatment.[2,4] Echinocandin medications are usually the first treatment recommendations for invasive candidiasis, but this is patient specific. Factors such as age, immune status, location, and severity of the infection are taken into account before treatment begins. Caspofungin, micafungin, anidulafungin, fluconazole, or amphotericin B may be given intravenously initially. Length of treatment is dependent

---

Table 4
Antifungal drug classifications

Antifungal Drug Class	Medications	Laboratory Monitoring	Nursing Considerations
Polyenes	Amphotericin B Liposomal amphotericin B Amphotericin B lipid complex	Monitor creatinine & BUN Monitor electrolytes Complete blood count Liver function tests	Premedication with antipyretics, antihistamines, or meperidine Infuse over 2–6 h Assess for nephrotoxicity and liver toxicity
Triazoles	Ketoconazole Itraconazole Fluconazole Voriconazole Posaconazole	Monitor blood levels Reduce does of fluconazole in patients with renal insufficiency	Increased drug interactions with cyclosporine, benzodiazepines, statins, and anti-HIV drugs
Novel agents • Echinocandins • Extended-spectrum triazoles	Caspofungin Micafungin Anidulafungin		Precautions with liver patients, pregnant patients, and those on cyclosporine

Data from Limper AH, Knox KS, Sarosi GA, et al. An official American Thoracic Society statement: treatment of fungal infections in adult pulmonary and critical care patients. Am J Respir Crit Care Med 2011;183:96–128.

Table 5
Treatment comparisons for specific fungal infections

Type of Treatment	Candida	Aspergillus	Cryptococcus	Histoplasmosis	P jirovecii	Coccidioidomycosis
Prophylaxis	Fluconazole Posaconazole	Posaconazole	n/a	n/a	n/a	n/a
Treatment	Capsofungin Micafungin	Voriconazole Micafungin	Fluconazole Amp. B	Amp. B Amp. B liposomal Fluconazole	TMP-SMX	Amp. B Fluconazole Itraconazole

Abbreviations: Amp. B, Amphotericin B; n/a, no recommendation; TMP-SMX, trimethoprim-sulfamethoxazole.

Data from Limper AH, Knox KS, Sarosi GA, et al. An official American Thoracic Society statement: treatment of fungal infections in adult pulmonary and critical care patients. Am J Respir Crit Care Med 2011;183:96–128; and Schmiedel Y, Zimmerli S. Common invasive fungal diseases: an overview of invasive candidiasis, aspergillosis, cryptococcosis, and pneumocystis pneumonia. Swiss Med Wkly 2016;146:w14281.

on the extent of the infection. The common treatment length is usually after signs and symptoms have dissipated or Candida is not found in the bloodstream.[2,4]

Caspofungin is primarily used for infections with Candida as is micafungin.[2,4] Furthermore, micafungin is used as prophylaxis against Candida infection in patients with stem cell transplant and those with Candida and Candida esophagitis.[2]

Aspergillus Management

Voriconazole is used for treatment of invasive aspergillus, whereas Itraconazole is effective with some aspergillus infections.[2] The Echinocandins, micafungin and anidulafungin, have activity against aspergillus.[2] Prophylaxis is recommended for patients receiving chemotherapy. Early treatment is necessary to ensure optimal patient outcomes and reduce the risk of morality. First-line treatments include azole medications. Treatments should be continued until all clinical signs and symptoms have resolved.[4]

Cryptococcus Management

Fluconazole has significant activity for the treatment of cryptococcus.[2] Although the clinical outcome in patients with fungal infections is poor and resistance to therapy is on the increase, new treatments are needed. The most common treatment is azole medications, such as posaconazole for cryptococcus.[16] Posaconazole is only available in oral suspension, which can be an issue in administration to critically ill patients. Combination therapies are often considered to include 2 antifungal medications to improve patient outcomes. In patients with cryptococcus, combination of amphotericin B plus an azole is often used. These are available in intravenous and oral formulations; some nursing considerations include the potential need for an inline filter or capsule, which cannot be opened for nasogastric tube administration. Flucytosine is commonly used to treat Cryptococcus[24]; treatment can be preemptive (those with high risk), prophylactic, or definitive treatment.[1]

Histoplasmosis Management

Asymptomatic infection may not require pharmacologic therapy, but treatment depends on expert opinion.[2] Amphotericin B is first-line therapy for severe fungal infections with histoplasmosis.[1,2] In patients taking multiple nephrotoxic drugs or existing renal insufficiency, a lipid form of amphotericin B has less effect on kidney function.[2] Itraconazole is effective for some histoplasmosis infections, but it has high protein binding and thus is not effective for central nervous system infections.

Pneumocystis jirovecii Pneumonia Management

Prophylaxis is indicated when CD4 counts are less than 200, patients are on cytotoxic drugs or chronic steroids, or the patient had an organ transplant.[1] The most effective treatment for severe pneumocystis pneumonia is trimethoprim-sulfamethoxazole.[2,4] Duration of therapy may vary from 3 weeks for HIV-positive patients to 14 days for non-HIV patients.[4] Caspofungin has some activity against pneumocystis.[2]

Coccidioidomycosis Management

Patients with pulmonary coccidioidomycosis are usually treated using the Infectious Disease Society of America guidelines using oral azoles as a first-line therapy.[2] Although ketoconazole is approved for use in coccidioidomycosis, fluconazole or itraconazole are widely used. Studies have supported a minimum dose of 400 mg of azoles; however, relapse after therapy is common.[2] Fluconazole has been shown to be most effective in treating coccidioidal meningitis. Patients with severe disseminated coccidioidomycosis are first treated with amphotericin B until symptom improvement and then followed by treatment with fluconazole or itraconazole for at least a year.[2]

SUMMARY

Fungal infections are increasing in critical care settings because more patients are immunocompromised from severe disease or medical treatments. Candida is the most frequently reported fungal infection, prompting the CDC to institute an Emerging Infection Program on Candida. Fatigue and fever are common presenting symptoms that require critical care nurses to remain vigilant in assessment to identify at-risk patients, promote use of timely cultures, and appropriate treatments for fungal infections. Critical care nurses can contribute to decreasing risk for fungal infections by controlling glucose levels, decreasing the use of invasive lines, and preventing unnecessary antibiotic use. More nursing research is needed to guide practice and track the incidence and prevalence of fungal infections in critical care.

REFERENCES

1. Bajwa SJ, Kulshrestha A. Fungal infections in intensive care unit: challenges in diagnosis and management. Ann Med Health Sci Res 2013;3:238–44.
2. Limper AH, Knox KS, Sarosi GA, et al. An official American Thoracic Society statement: treatment of fungal infections in adult pulmonary and critical care patients. Am J Respir Crit Care Med 2011;183:96–128.
3. Chen SC, Sorrell TC, Chang CC, et al. Consensus guidelines for the treatment of yeast infections in the haematology, oncology and intensive care setting. Intern Med J 2014;44:1315–25.
4. Schmiedel Y, Zimmerli S. Common invasive fungal diseases: an overview of invasive candidiasis, aspergillosis, cryptococcosis, and pneumocystis pneumonia. Swiss Med Wkly 2016;146:w14281.
5. van Vught LA, Klein PMC, Spitoni C, et al. Incidence, risk factors, and attributable mortality of secondary infections in the intensive care unit after admission for sepsis. JAMA 2016;315(5):1469–78.
6. CDC. Invasive candidiasis page. 2015. Available at: http://www.cdc.gov/fungal/diseases/candidiasis/invasive/statistics.html. Accessed August 21, 2016.
7. CDC. Emerging infections program—healthcare-associated infections projects page. 2016. Available at: http://www.cdc.gov/hai/eip/candida.html. Accessed August 21, 2016.
8. Vila J, Martinez JA. Opportunistic infections in the intensive care unit: a microbiologic overview. In: Rello J, Kollef M, Diaz E, et al, editors. Infectious diseases in critical care. 2nd edition. Heidelberg (Germany); Berlin: Springer; 2007. p. 29–34. Available at: http://link.springer.com/chapter/10.1007%2F978-3-540-34406-3_4#page-1. Accessed August 25, 2016.
9. Magill SS, Edwards JR, Bamberg W, et al. Multistate point-prevalence survey of health care-associated infections. N Engl J Med 2014;370:1198–208.
10. CDC. Aspergillosis statistics page. 2015. Available at: http://www.cdc.gov/fungal/diseases/aspergillosis/statistics.html. Accessed August 21, 2016.
11. CDC. C. Gattii infection statistics page. 2015. Available at: http://www.cdc.gov/fungal/diseases/cryptococcosis-gattii/statistics.html. Accessed August 21, 2016.
12. CDC. C. Neoformans infection statistics page. 2015. Available at: http://www.cdc.gov/fungal/diseases/cryptococcosis-neoformans/statistics.html. Accessed August 21, 2016.

13. CDC. Histoplasmosis statistics page. Available at: http://www.cdc.gov/fungal/diseases/histoplasmosis/statistics.html Updated February 8, 2016. Accessed August 21, 2016.
14. CDC. Pneumocystis pneumonia page. 2014. Available at: http://www.cdc.gov/fungal/diseases/pneumocystis-pneumonia/. Accessed August 21, 2016.
15. CDC. Valley fever (coccidioidomycosis) statistics page. 2016. Available at: http://www.cdc.gov/fungal/diseases/coccidioidomycosis/statistics.html. Accessed August 21, 2016.
16. Zaragoza O, Rodrigues M, DeJesus M, et al. The capsule of the fungal pathogen cryptococcus neoformans. Adv Appl Microbiol 2009;68:133–216.
17. CDC. Coccidioidomycosis health care professionals page. 2016. Available at: http://www.cdc.gov/fungal/diseases/coccidioidomycosis/health-professionals.html. Accessed September 1, 2016.
18. Ferry D. The fever. Mother Jones 2015;40(1):30–9.
19. Patolia S, Kennedy E, Zahir M, et al. Risk factors for candida blood stream infection in medical ICU and role of colonization—a retrospective study. Br J Med Pract 2013;6(1):a618.
20. CDC. Candida health care professionals page. 2016. Available at: http://www.cdc.gov/fungal/diseases/candidiasis/invasive/health-professionals.html. Accessed September 1, 2016.
21. Beed M, Sherman R, Holden S. Fungal infections and critically ill adults. Contin Educ Anaesth Crit Care Pain 2014;14(6):262–7.
22. Taccone F, Van den Abeele A, Bulpa P, et al. Epidemiology of invasive aspergillosis in critically ill patients: clinical presentation, underlying conditions and outcomes. Crit Care 2015;19:7.
23. Vallabhanei S, Haselow D, Lloyd S, et al. Cluster of Cryptococcus neoformans infections in intensive care unit. Emerg Infect Dis 2015;21:1719–24.
24. Groth C, Dodds-Ashley E. Fungal infections in the ICU. Infection in critical care. CCSAP 2016 book 1. Norwell (MA): Kluwer Academic Publishers; 2016.
25. Capriotti T, Frizzell JP. Infectious diseases. In: Capriotti T, Frizzell JP, editors. Pathophysiology introductory concepts and clinical perspectives. Philadelphia: F.A. Davis Company; 2016. p. 194–6.
26. Kim SJ, Lee J, Cho YJ, et al. Prognostic factors of Pneumocystis jirovecii pneumonia in patients without HIV infection. J Infect 2014;69:88–95.
27. Li MC, Lee NY, Lee CC, et al. Pneumocystis jiroveci pneumonia in immunocompromised patients: delayed diagnosis and poor outcomes in non-HIV-infected individuals. J Microbiol Immunol Infect 2014;47:42–7.

Wound Infections in Critical Care

Jean E. Cefalu, PhD, APRN, AGNP-C, CWOCN, CFCN, CNE[a],*, Kendra M. Barrier, PhD, RN, MSN[b],
Alison H. Davis, PhD, RN, CHSE[c]

KEYWORDS

- Wound healing • Evidence-based nursing • Wound management • Wound infection
- Critical care nursing

KEY POINTS

- Antimicrobial resistance rates in the critical care environment are higher because of the widespread use of broad-spectrum antibiotics, multiple invasive procedures, and transmission of multiple drug–resistant bacteria between patients.
- Clinical signs and symptoms of wound colonization and infection share similarities and can be difficult to differentiate.
- Nurses must be adept at distinguishing normal wound drainage from the initial inflammatory response from an overt infectious process.
- Biofilms form rapidly in wounds given the right environment, delay wound healing by competing for metabolic resources, and prolong the inflammatory phase.
- Numerous commercially available antimicrobial/antiseptic agents have been developed and should be considered as part of a comprehensive wound management strategy.

Patients admitted to critical care units are at high risk for increase morbidity and mortality from skin and deep wound infections. Antimicrobial resistance rates are higher because of the widespread use of broad-spectrum antibiotics, multiple invasive procedures, and transmission of multiple drug–resistant bacteria between patients.[1,2] *Staphylococcus aureus* is part of the normal skin flora found on 20% to 50% of healthy adults. In hospitals, *S aureus* is the major cause of acute bacterial skin and skin structure infections, especially surgical site infections.[3] *S aureus* isolates increased from 35,553 isolates in 1996 to 190,654 isolates in 2008 in United States hospitals, a ~5.4-fold increase.[4] Methicillin-resistant *S aureus* (MRSA) isolates accounted for

[a] Nursing Department, School of Nursing, Louisiana State University Health Sciences Center, 1900 Gravier Street, Suite 4A6, New Orleans, LA 70112, USA; [b] School of Nursing, Louisiana State University Health Sciences Center, 1900 Gravier Street, Suite 4C1, New Orleans, LA 70112, USA; [c] School of Nursing, Louisiana State University Health Sciences Center, 1900 Gravier Street, Suite 506, New Orleans, LA 70112, USA
* Corresponding author.
E-mail address: jeric1@lsuhsc.edu

Crit Care Nurs Clin N Am 29 (2017) 81–96
http://dx.doi.org/10.1016/j.cnc.2016.09.009
ccnursing.theclinics.com
0899-5885/17/© 2016 Elsevier Inc. All rights reserved.

53% of all *S aureus* isolates in US hospitals from 2006 to 2008 with more than half cultured in the critical care environment.[4] Prevention, early recognition, and management of wound infections are critical to successful outcomes in this patient population. This article addresses the physiologic basis for wound healing and the complexities of the wound microenvironment, distinguishing inflammation from infection, recognition of biofilms, and evidence-based wound management guidelines to promote wound healing.

PHYSIOLOGIC BASIS FOR WOUND HEALING
Skin Anatomy and Physiology

The skin is the human body's largest organ and the first line of defense from environmental insults (**Box 1**). The skin and its appendages (eccrine glands, apocrine glands, and hair follicles) make up this complex organ system. Although the distribution of appendages and skin thickness vary depending on the location, the basic structural components remain constant.[5] Human skin is divided into 2 layers: a superficial epidermal layer generally about 0.04 mm thick, and a deeper connective tissue layer called the dermis. The epidermis and dermis overlay the hypodermis, a layer of subcutaneous fat tissue containing large blood vessels that supply the skin and play a crucial role in thermoregulation and pressure redistribution.[5–7] The epidermis of human skin is a living ecosystem colonized by more than 10^3 microorganisms (per gram of tissue) including bacteria, fungi, and viruses.[8] These symbiotic microorganisms provide protection against invasion and overgrowth of more pathogenic organisms.

The epidermis is a stratified epithelium composed of 4 layers over most of the body and a fifth layer (stratum lucidum) of translucent cells found on the palms of the hands and soles of the feet. Keratinocytes are the primary cells in the epidermis. The stratum basale or stratum germinativum is the deepest layer of the epidermis and attaches to the dermis by an adhesive basement membrane. The basement membrane is the layer involved in blister formation.[9] A single layer of mitotically active keratinocytes forms the stratum basale and is responsible for all epidermal regeneration. When the epidermis is injured, cell division in the basal layer greatly accelerates. As new cells form, older cells migrate toward the skin surface through the stratum spinosum and stratum granulosum, undergoing terminal differentiation by the time they reach the outermost layer, the stratum corneum.[9]

The stratum corneum is made up of 20 to 30 layers of dead keratinocytes, which provides a protective, durable overcoat that is tough, waterproof, and fairly insensitive to biological, chemical, and physical assault. Normal skin is slightly acidic (5.5 pH) and the layered keratinocytes and lipids of the epidermis form the acid mantle that inhibits microbial growth. Underneath the surface, immune cells, including polymorphonuclear neutrophils, Langerhans cells, and macrophages, destroy pathogenic

---

Box 1
Skin functions

- Protection
- Prevention of fluid loss
- Thermoregulation
- Sensation
- Synthesis of vitamin D

microorganisms in the dermis. Langerhans cells are scattered throughout the epidermal and dermal layers. These specialized macrophages provide the first immunologic barrier to the external environment.[8–10]

The dermis consists of 2 layers: the papillary dermis and the deeper reticular dermis. The papillary dermis consists of loosely woven fibers embedded in an extracellular matrix (ECM) and fibroblasts (collagen production), ground substance, and elastin that provide tensile strength (turgor and toughness). The fibroblasts secrete fibronectin and hyaluronic acid thought to have important biological roles in wound healing.[10] The reticular dermis is thicker and composed of interconnecting collagen bundles and large elastic fibers within a viscous gel rich in mucopolysaccharides. Collagen fibers are organized into bundles that run parallel to the body's surface and underlying muscle fibers, which provide tensile strength[7,9] Langer lines are topological map lines that correspond with the natural orientation of collagen fibers in the dermis. Surgical incisions are often determined by the organizational pattern of the Langer lines because of minimal disruption of the fibers and decreased scarring.[11]

Wound Microenvironment

The ECM is the epicenter of wound healing. The intricate meshwork of macromolecules constituting the ECM is not only critical for connecting cells together to form tissue but provides the substrate on which cell migration is guided during wound healing. The ECM is responsible for the relay of environmental signals to the surfaces of individual cells. The 2 main classes of molecules in the ECM are fibrous proteins (collagen, elastin, fibronectin, and laminin) and glycosaminoglycans (GAGs). The high viscosity and low compressibility of GAGs provides the structural integrity of the cells and lubricates the passageways between cells, allowing cell migration. The combination of the ECM, fibroblasts, and ground substance makes up connective tissue.[8]

Wound Healing

Partial-thickness and full-thickness wounds heal through 4 well-orchestrated phases: hemostasis, inflammation, proliferation, and remodeling. Hemostasis occurs immediately after injury to minimize blood loss. During hemostasis, blood vessels constrict and platelets activate by binding to exposed collagen in the ECM. The platelets secrete fibronectin, thrombospondin, sphingosine 1 phosphate, and von Willebrand factor, which promote platelet activation and aggregation. The resulting fibrin matrix deposits in the wound to form a stable clot and seals off lymphatic flow to prevent infection. In addition to clot formation, platelets secrete cytokines and growth factors including platelet-derived growth factor (PDGF) and transforming growth factor beta (TGF-β) that signal neutrophils and fibroblasts to the site of injury.[5]

The inflammatory phase begins within the first 24 hours, characterized by redness, heat, swelling, and pain from the release of vasoactive amines and histamine from the mast cells. Histamine released from the mast cells causes surrounding vessels to leak fluid, which promotes the movement of neutrophils, macrophages, and lymphocytes from the vessels to the site of injury. Neutrophils phagocytize bacteria, foreign materials, and other cellular debris. As neutrophils die, they release the intracellular enzyme elastase, which promotes further digestion of devitalized tissue. Macrophages provide a second line of defense and secrete matrix-degrading enzymes and matrix metalloproteases to facilitate movement through the wound and break down devitalized tissue at the wound site. Macrophages also secrete several growth factors, including PDGF and TGF-β, that facilitate wound progression to the proliferative phase.[12–15]

The proliferative phase usually overlaps the inflammatory phase and is characterized by the formation of new blood vessels (angiogenesis), granulation tissue (in wounds healing by secondary or tertiary intention), and epithelization. Endothelial cells support the regeneration of damaged capillary beds. Fibroblasts produce the collagen and GAGs needed for the formation of granulation tissue. Healthy granulation tissue appears red, described as beefy buds, with wet sugar crystals in an open wound. Granulation tissue contains macrophages, fibroblasts, immature collagen, blood vessels, and ground substance. Epidermal migration is the final step in the proliferative phase. During epithelialization, keratinocytes migrate inward from the edges of the wound until they meet, sealing off the wound surface.[15]

The final maturation or remodeling phase can last from 21 days to years depending on several host factors, including age, nutritional status, and comorbid chronic disease states that have an effect on metabolism, oxygenation, or perfusion. During this phase, type III collagen is replaced with stronger type I collagen and fibers reorganize to increase tensile strength. Note that scar tissue only regains 80% of normal tissue strength and therefore is always at risk for repeated injury or breakdown.[14,15]

INFLAMMATION VERSUS INFECTION

Immediately after a breach in the skin's surface, both normal flora and pathogenic organisms contaminate the wound bed. This warm, moist, nutrient-rich subepidermal environment provides a rich medium for pathogenic organisms to replicate and thrive.

Infection is therefore a common complication in any type of wound. Systemic signs of infection in acute or chronic wounds may present with fever, increased white blood cell count, and red lines streaking away from the wound representing progression of the infection into the lymphatic system. Clinical signs and symptoms of wound colonization and infection share similarities and thus can be difficult to differentiate. Inflammation is an innate protective immune response necessary to remove offending pathogens. Inflammation is not diagnostic of infection. Clinicians must be adept at distinguishing normal wound drainage from the initial inflammatory response and from an overt infectious process. **Table 1** compares signs and symptoms of inflammation versus infection.

Immunocompromised patients may or may not show the classic signs and symptoms of inflammation or infection.[13] Confirming wound infection is generally done by colony count. Colony counts higher than 100,000 (10^5) organisms per gram of tissue or per milliliter of fluid are considered confirmation of an infection.[16,17]

Bioburden

Bioburden refers to the amount or load of microorganisms in a wound. Once the skin barrier is breached, the wound surface is immediately contaminated with planktonic (free-floating) nonreplicating skin flora as well as any opportunistic bacteria, fungi, and viruses that were in close proximity to the site of injury. The presence of bacteria in a wound is beneficial because it initiates the inflammatory response needed to begin healing.[17] Bacterial colonization refers to the presence of replicating bacteria on the wound surface. Contaminated and colonized wounds do not show invasion or damage to nearby tissue and do not stimulate a host immune response. Contaminated and colonized wounds should be monitored for the development of infection but seldom interfere with wound healing.[5,18]

The term critical colonization was developed in an attempt to explain the critical role bacteria play in the failure of wounds to heal as expected. Critical colonization indicates replicating bacteria impeding wound healing without signs of an acute inflammation (pain, erythema, induration, edema, increased exudate, or warmth).[18] Critical colonization is frequently referred to as a local infection. Wounds that stop progressing

Table 1
Signs and symptoms of inflammation versus infection

Sign or Symptom	Inflammation	Infection
Erythema	Well-defined borders, mild to moderate redness. Sometimes difficult to assess in darker skin tones (use the back of the hand to assess for warmth)	Intense redness, distinct borders, >0.5 cm extension from the wound, red streaking may appear proximal to and distal from the wound
Induration/edema	Firmness at wound edge and mild edema from increased capillary permeability	Firmness spreading out from wound edge and increasing edema
Exudate	Odor subsides after cleansing and removal of necrotic tissue and dressing debris. Minimal exudate that subsides over 3–5 d. Usually sanguineous, serosanguineous, or serous	Odor remains after removal of necrotic tissue and dressing debris. Moderate to heavy amounts of seropurulent to purulent exudate noted or a sudden increase in exudate • Pseudomonas: sweet • Proteus: ammonia
Pain	Variable depending on the degree of inflammation. Increases then gradually subsides	Persistent and continues for an extended amount of time or increase in pain
Systemic fever	Usually absent	Usually present unless immunocompromised
White blood cell count	Usually normal	Increased
Granulation tissue	Red beefy buds of tissue	Friable; bleeds easily

toward healing, show a noticeable difference in the quality or quantity of granulation tissue, and show an increase in the amount of exudate are considered or assumed to be critically colonized.[18,19] Critical colonization is suspected based on clinical characteristics and not quantifiable biomarkers such as bacterial loads less than 100,000 colony-forming units per gram of tissue. The presence of critical colonization is supported by a positive response to topical antibiotics or use of an antimicrobial dressing.[19] The concept of critical colonization helps to explain biofilm development in chronic wounds.[20–23]

Biofilms

Biofilm formation is a serious problem frequently occurring in chronic wounds,[24] but can occur in an acute wound given the right conditions. Biofilms have been implicated in more than 80% of device-related surgical site infections.[20,25] Biofilms develop when microorganisms attach to the wound surface and begin to replicate. Biofilms can develop from 1 bacterial species but are generally formed with multiple species of bacteria as well as yeast and fungi. The new microbial community interacts in a stable symbiotic relationship to produce an extracellular polymeric substance consisting of water, polysaccharides, proteins, glycolipids, and extracellular DNA.[26] This gelatinous matrix makes bacteria living within the biofilm almost impervious to antiseptics, antibiotics, phagocytic neutrophils, macrophages, and displacement. Biofilms are considerably more difficult to remove than planktonic bacteria.[20,23] Biofilms form rapidly in wounds given the right environment, delay wound healing by competing for metabolic resources, and prolong the inflammatory phase.[26] Research suggests that traditional culture methods may not be adequate in detecting biofilm composition.[27,28]

Infection

Acute bacterial skin infections are predominantly cause by aerobic gram-positive cocci, most notably beta-hemolytic streptococci and S aureus.[29,30] In contrast, chronic wounds are often contaminated with species of normal skin flora and occasionally gram-negative organisms.[30] The most common skin and wound contaminants are listed in **Table 2**.

QUANTITATIVE WOUND CULTURE

Quantitative wound cultures are recommended to confirm infection, isolate microbes, and guide therapy. The best techniques for obtaining wound cultures remain the subject of considerable debate.[31] The proper technique is to capture bacteria in live tissue, not bacteria on the wound surface, or from necrotic tissue. Tissue biopsy, needle aspiration of wound fluid, curettage, and quantitative swabs are the most used in clinical practice. All are used to test for both aerobic and anaerobic microbes.

Tissue Biopsy

Tissue biopsy is the removal of a small sample of tissue using a scalpel or punch. Tissue biopsy has been advocated as the gold standard for wound culture where infection is suspected.[31,32] Although tissue biopsy is the gold standard, it is an invasive procedure, often painful, and costly, and must be performed by qualified and trained providers whose schedules are unpredictable. Therefore, tissue biopsies are not commonly used.[32,33]

Tissue or punch biopsies are appropriate in the critical care setting because of the severity of illness. Copeland-Halperin and colleagues[31] conducted a systematic review to evaluate the evidence for using a swab culture compared with tissue biopsy. Moderate-quality evidence showed that punch biopsies provided qualitative and quantitative information on bacterial load with nearly 100% sensitivity, 90% specificity, and 95% accuracy for predicting wound closure.

A deep tissue biopsy should be performed after initial debridement and cleaning of superficial debris with an antiseptic-free, sterile solution. To minimize pain, the biopsy area should be treated with a topical or local anesthetic. Pressure is applied to the biopsy area to control bleeding after the sample is obtained. Biopsy samples should be transported to the laboratory immediately.

Needle aspiration involves insertion of a needle into the tissue to aspirate fluid containing microbes. The skin of the periwound should be cleansed with a disinfectant

Table 2
The most common skin and wound contaminants

Aerobes	Anaerobes
S aureus	Bacteroides spp
Staphylococcus epidermidis	Fusobacterium spp
Streptococcus pyogenes	Peptostreptococcus spp
Pseudomonas aeruginosa	Veillonella spp
MRSA	Porphyromonas spp
Enterococcus faecalis	
Coliforms	
Acinetobacter baumannii	

and allowed to dry. A 10-mL syringe with 0.5 mL of air predrawn and a 22-gauge needle are needed. The needle is inserted through intact skin with suction applied by pulling back on the plunger to the 10-mL mark. The needle is moved in and out at different angles 2 to 4 times and then withdrawn, capped, and sent to the laboratory.[33]

Curettage is the surgical removal of wound tissue using a spoon-shaped instrument called a curette. Curettage can isolate anaerobic bacteria and disrupts biofilm at the same time, giving curettage an advantage compared with other quantitative techniques. The procedure uses a 3-mm curette with a single scraping from the edge or undermined area of a wound. The scraping should harvest at least 20 mg of tissue for analysis. Curettage is used in maintenance debridement of chronic wounds and is effective in opening a short therapeutic window for disruption and weakening of biofilms. Curettage is less invasive than tissue biopsy and has shown higher sensitivity and specificity than quantitative swab cultures.[34]

Quantitative Swab

Wound swabs are minimally invasive, easy to perform, and widely used in clinical practice, but vary in technique. In comparative studies, the Levine technique (**Box 2**) was superior to the Z-swab technique.[31,35] Biopsies have shown greater sensitivity and specificity than swab cultures. Current evidence suggests that swabs may be useful for initial wound monitoring, whereas biopsies are preferred when antibiotic resistance is suspected.[34,35]

The Levine technique has been shown to identify more organisms in acute wounds and chronic wounds compared with other swab techniques.[35,36] The Levine technique showed higher diagnostic accuracy compared with the Z technique and both the Levine technique and the Z technique showed higher diagnostic accuracy than tissue biopsy.[31,35,37]

Box 2
Levine wound swab culture technique

1. Follow standard precautions for infection control.

2. Always obtain the culture from properly cleaned and prepared tissue to avoid surface contamination.

3. Obtain appropriate Culturette supplies: 2-swab system for aerobes and Gram stains and 1-swab system for anaerobes.

4. Collect the culture before initiation of topical or systemic antibiotics.

5. Obtain the swab culture from a viable (living) wound bed; do not culture necrotic tissue or wound exudate.

6. Irrigate the wound with normal saline and wipe the surface vigorously with sterile gauze moistened with preservative-free sterile saline.

7. Blot excess saline from the wound bed.

8. Moisten the swab with normal saline if the wound bed is dry (soaking dilutes the sample).

9. Rotate the swab over a 1-cm to 2-cm area of viable tissue with enough force to produce exudate and return the applicator to the Culturette.

10. Transport immediately to the laboratory (<2 hours) after collection.

Data from Levine NS, Lindberg RB, Mason AD, et al. The quantitative swab culture and smear: a quick simple method for determining the number of viable aerobic bacteria on open wounds. J Trauma 1976;16(2):89–94; Bonham PA. Swab cultures for diagnosing wound infections: a literature review and clinical guideline. J Wound Ostomy Continence Nurs 2009;36(4):389–95.

Management of Exudate and Infection

Treatment of wound infections in critical care units represents a great challenge, especially those caused by gram-negative organisms.

Treatment of infection should first focus on optimizing the patient's overall health status by addressing underlying medical conditions, such as nutrition, circulation, oxygenation, and management of chronic disease such as diabetes.[5,16] Systemic antibiotics are not always necessary and are addressed elsewhere in this issue.

Local management of wound infections includes debridement to remove necrotic tissue, wound cleansing, and the use of topical antibiotics and appropriate secondary dressings.

The key principles of topical management of wound infection correspond with the essential elements needed to establish a wound environment that supports healing (moisture balance, control of bioburden, temperature control, and regulation of pH).

Debridement

Adequate preparation of the wound bed begins with an assessment of wound tissue. Necrotic tissue delays wound healing, mechanically obstructs wound contraction, perpetuates the inflammatory process, and provides a fertile environment for bacterial replication. Once adequate blood flow is confirmed (particularly on a distal extremity), removal of necrotic tissue can be done by surgical, conservative sharp, enzymatic, larval, or autolytic methods. Mechanical debridement such as wet-to-dry dressings are extremely painful and damage newly formed granulation tissue. Wet-to-dry dressings do not promote wound healing, are expensive, and therefore should be avoided.[38-40]

Surgical debridement is recommended for wounds with advancing cellulitis, wound-related sepsis, and/or infected bone or hardware that must be removed.[41] Surgical debridement is the most efficient method of removing large amounts of necrotic tissue (skin, fat, fascia, bone, muscle, and tendon) and living tissue (nonselective) down to a healthy wound base, and restarts the wound healing process in stalled wounds. Risk must be considered, patients are likely to need anesthesia, and there is a potential for bleeding and infection. This method should only be performed by a skilled surgeon.

Conservative sharp debridement is used in the presence of loosely adherent necrotic tissue where necrotic tissue can be selectively removed with the use of sterile instruments, including scalpel, forceps, and scissors. The debridement is confined to necrotic tissue with no anticipated blood loss, therefore it is considered low risk. The conservative debridement method requires an experienced practitioner, knowledgeable of anatomy and resources, to manage complications of bleeding or infection. Conservative sharp debridements are typically done in conjunction with other debridement methods and/or with each dressing change.

Enzymatic debridement is a method of removing necrotic tissue with the topical application of enzymes to degrade collagen. Collagenase is the only enzymatic debridement agent available in the United States.[42,43] Collagenase digests the denatured collagen that anchors the tissue to the underlying wound bed. Collagenase is safe for use in infected wounds and with selected topical antibiotics and antibacterial dressings. However, collagenase is inactivated in the presence of iodine and many silver-based products.[43] Compared with other debridement methods, enzymatic debridement is expensive, slow, and has shown efficacy compared with autolysis. Some studies have reported enzymatic debridement to be cost-effective.[42,43] Treatment should continue until all necrotic tissue is removed and then discontinued. Collagenase must be applied daily and requires increased nursing time. The cost associated with daily dressing changes must be considered.[44]

Larval (maggot) therapy has been used since the Civil War, before the introduction of antibiotics, and is a quick and efficient method for removing slough and debris from wounds. Sterile *Lucilia sericata* (green bottle fly) larvae are applied, which secrete powerful enzymes to break down necrotic tissue without destroying healthy granulation tissue. Many patients and nurses find this method distasteful, therefore larval therapy has declined since the 1940s. Larval therapy remains an option for patients with infected wounds and patients who are not surgical candidates. Research has not found larval therapy to be more effective than other debridement methods.[45,46]

Autolytic debridement is the natural process that involves the breakdown of necrotic tissue by the body's normal inflammatory process. Proteolytic, fibrinolytic, and collagenolytic enzymes selectively digest necrotic tissue, leaving healthy tissue intact. Autolytic debridement is considered safe, slow, and effective, but is not used on infected wounds.[47] Many dressings that provide a warm moist environment support autolytic debridement (transparent film, polyacrylate, hydrogels, and medical grade honey). During the early phases of autolytic debridement, frequent dressing changes may be needed because of liquefaction of the slough and other debris. In addition, the periwound needs to be protected from maceration and degradation by application of an impervious skin barrier (skin prep). Nurses should assess the wound for signs of infection with every dressing change, keeping in mind that increased exudate is expected during autolytic debridement.

Wound Cleansing

Cleansing the wound bed is the next step in preparing for wound healing. There is a general agreement that all wounds should be cleansed with each dressing change, before and after debridement, and if contaminated from urine or stool.[47–50] The universally recommended solution for wound cleansing is 0.9% isotonic saline (normal saline) used in conjunction with enough pressure (4–15 pounds per square inch [psi]) to mechanically clean, remove loosely adherent contaminants, and devitalize tissue from the wound surface, without driving bacteria deeper into the surrounding tissue.[47] Normal saline is cost-effective, most widely used, and safe for all cell types, but is not bacteriostatic or bactericidal. The most recent Cochrane systematic review failed to find evidence to support the benefits of healing or infection control with the use of sterile normal saline compared with potable tap water in acute or chronic wounds.[48] In a double-blind randomized controlled clinical trial, Weiss and colleagues[50] found tap water to be just as safe and effective as sterile normal saline.

The selection of a cleanser is guided by the wound characteristics. Topical solutions are toxic to fibroblasts, therefore consideration is needed. There is weak evidence for the recommendations to use noncytotoxic solutions, combined with mechanical force to remove surface debris without injuring newly developed tissue and driving bacteria deeper into the wound.[41] Commercially available wound cleaners have an advantage of having calibrated pumps to deliver 11 psi. A daily pulsatile lavage of 11 psi was shown to have an advantage compared with low-psi or no-pressure wound lavage.[49]

Current research focuses on techniques and the composition of cleaning fluids rather than the physiologic processes that take place. In 1992, Angeras and colleagues[51] conducted a quasirandomized study that alternately assigned adult postoperative patients sutured less than 6 hours after injury to cleansing with tap water at 37°C (n = 295) or room temperature saline (21°C; n = 322). Results showed that warm tap water was more effective than nonwarmed saline in reducing the infection rate. Solutions should be warmed to body temperature. Cleansing a wound with products at room temperature versus warmed products results in local vasoconstriction, halting wound healing for up to 40 minutes with each dressing change.[52]

Vasoconstriction limits oxygen concentrations in the wound, impairs immune function, and promotes bacterial replication.[53] Therefore, clinicians should take the time to warm wound cleansers before application.

Topical Antibiotics

Wounds do not have to be sterile to heal. Wounds can continue to heal in the presence of clinical infection, negating the use of topical antibiotics for routine skin infections. One exception is the use of topical metronidazole to control odor in malodourous and fungating wounds. Although topical antibiotics have fewer adverse effects, local allergic reactions and resistant organisms may emerge with widespread and prolonged use. As discussed previously, the use of topical antibiotics may be of limited value in the presence of biofilms and in the presence of advancing infections. Systemic antibiotic therapy is warranted in these situations.[41]

Antimicrobial Wound Dressings

Commercially available antimicrobial/antiseptic dressings provide consistent, broad-spectrum activity and serve as an additional treatment modality. In certain conditions, these antimicrobial dressing are an addition to systemic antibiotic therapy or provide sufficient therapy independently. These agents provide a physical barrier to potential contaminants while interacting with exudate, if present, thus reducing the bacterial load of a wound. These dressings have been reported to be easy to use, comfortable, and conformable; to provide visualization of the wound; and to avoid additional pain on removal.[54,55]

Antimicrobials/antiseptics act on multiple sites within bacteria, which may explain low levels of resistance. This multiple-site phenomenon allows topical antiseptics to be considered as appropriate to use in immunocompromised patients to prevent wounds or in wounds with nonmodifiable patient factors or systemic factors. To date, most antiseptics are considered as toxic to fibroblasts at typical concentrations, so their use remains controversial.

Toxic effects of antiseptics have been shown to be dose dependent. This finding is most evident with hydrogen peroxide and hypochlorous acid (HOCl). These agents were previously thought to be cytotoxic and are now showing efficacy in low concentrations.[24,56] In a quasirandomized controlled trial, Mohammadi and colleagues[56] were able to show beneficial effects of 2% hydrogen peroxide in decreasing bioburden in chronically colonized burn wounds. Significant improvement ($P<.05$) in burn graft take was found between limbs treated for 5 minutes with 2% hydrogen peroxide compared with limbs treated with sterile normal saline.

Hypochlorous acid

HOCl can be organic or inorganic. HOCl is a highly effective bactericidal compound. Cellular death has been noted against all bacterial, viral, and fungal human pathogens. Small amounts of HOCl solution have been shown to kill spore-forming and non–spore-forming bacteria as well as to destroy biofilms produced by numerous microorganisms. Antimicrobial rates have been reported from 0 minutes to 5 minutes after application of HOCl.[24] Organic HOCl is produced by white blood cells, neutrophils, in response to bound microorganisms, leading to increased cellular permeability.[57,58] Wang and colleagues[59] synthesized HOCl through the acidification of hypochlorite, resulting in a pH range of 3.5 to 4.0 for infection control. This synthetization resulted in a physiologically balanced solution with the potential to control wound infections.[59] At present, there is a lack of variety of HOCl applications, other than solutions, which may lessen the practicality of HOCl. Further studies are warranted.

Sodium hypochlorite
Sodium hypochlorite solutions have been used in wound care applications for hundreds of years and are as familiar to practitioners as Dakin solution (NaOCl). In the last 15 years, more advanced HOCl solutions, based on electrochemistry, have emerged as safe and viable wound-cleansing agents and infection treatment adjunct therapies. However, recommendations of the World Union of Wound Healing Societies (WUWHS) noted that the supporting evidence for the effectiveness of sodium hypochlorite is limited and do not recommend the routine use of this solution.[60] Additional research is warranted.

Silver
Silver is another agent with centuries of use because of its bactericidal properties in low concentrations with low risk of toxicity to human cells. As with other historical agents, advancements in wound care have resulted in numerous delivery methods for silver, including amorphous and sheet hydrogels, alginates, hydrofibers, foams, powders, foams, and irrigants.[54,55] O'Neill and colleagues[61] and Sibbald and colleagues[62] indicated that silver creams were most effective against bacteria. While contained in a dressing, silver acts by causing death of an organism on surfaces through donation to the wound bed or remains in dressings where it functions as a bactericidal agent to exudate. Overall, the ionized form of silver causes rapid, enduring bacterial cell death, thus decreasing wound infections.[5] However, the release of silver must be controlled in a time-release system in order to prevent toxicity to tissues and resulting in mucilaginous slough.[5,60–62] In large wounds, the use of a silver dressing has been associated with systemic toxicity and should be used with caution. The use of silver is contraindicated in combination with collagenase, as previously discussed.[44]

Honey
Honey has historical context, with accounts of honey-based wound healing noted in ancient times.[63] The use of honey for wound healing decreased with the invention of antibiotics, but has begun a resurgence because of antibiotic resistance.[64] Associated with wound care and healing, honey has been transformed into a medical grade, bacteria-inhibiting, acidic, and enzymatic activity–laden product of modern wound care practitioners. These properties provide the therapeutic effects of honey, including antiinflammatory effects, antibacterial effects, debridement abilities, and odor control. Medical grade honey is found in alginate, hydrocolloid, and paste form, in which it has antimicrobial effects against viruses, fungi, protozoa, and a multitude of bacteria. Pieper[63] reports a honey dressing product as approved by the United States Food and Drug Administration in 2007. The wound healing effects of honey are inconclusive in the literature, with reports of shortened healing time, infection eradication without systemic antibiotics, and decreased scarring.[63] Asamoah and colleagues[64] reported inconclusive results regarding the healing effects of honey.[63] The lack of randomized controlled studies contributes to the contradictory results.

Precautions must be taken if there are reports of persistent stinging or burning after initial application. These reported side effects are uncommon, but negate the use of an alternate antimicrobial wound dressing to promote patient comfort and safety. Contraindications include an allergy to honey and/or known allergy to bee products or stings.[54,55]

Gentian violet and methylene blue
Gentian violet and methylene blue are a combination used for 50 years as a bacteriostatic antiseptic. Recent advances in the delivery of gentian violet and methylene blue

include the ability to have these agents available in a polyvinyl alcohol (PVA) foam, wound packing, and ostomy rings. PVA can include silver for a combination effect. Benefits of PVA as a delivery method include exudate absorbability (12 times the foam's weight), reduction of rolled wound edges because of its conformability, compatibility with collagenase, and sensitivity to the wound bed when removed.[44,65] The combination of gentian violet and methylene blue in the foam dressing acts to trap and inhibit bacterial division, which minimizes the bacterial count in the host. The lack of bacterial division is associated with an increase in the proliferative stage of healing for the patient.[65] Gentian violet and methylene blue dressings are compatible with enzymatic debriding agents such as collagenase.[44,65]

Dialkylcarbamoylchloride

Dialkylcarbamoylchloride (DACC) does not deliver chemicals or antimicrobials to wound beds. These dressings remove bacteria physically through binding of bacteria. As the bacteria are bound to the layer of hydrophobic fatty acid derivative located on the contact layer of the dressing, bacteria become inactive and are removed with dressing changes.[54,55] The key to these dressings is the moisture level because bacteria attach to the dressing via moisture. Therefore, the use of additional antiseptics and analgesics is contraindicated because the moisture balance for adherence may be disturbed. Considerations with DACC include frequent dressing changes in wounds with signs of bacterial colonization or infection; this may necessitate frequent dressing changes as twice a day or daily because the goal is the physical removal of bacteria. However, DACC dressings have the ability to remain in place for up to 2 weeks when minimal exudate is present. In cases of excessive exudate, a secondary dressing with absorptive properties should be used in conjunction with DACC.

Polyhexamethylene biguanide

Polyhexamethylene biguanide (PHMB) has no known resistance and can be applied in a variety of applications because of its nontoxic characteristics. However, PHMB is not recommended for the primary treatment of active wound infections because of the agent's necessity to have direct contact with bacterial organisms.[54,55] However, when used in conjunction with a barrier dressing, PHMB impairs both infiltration and growth of pathogens into wounds. Practitioners should evaluate the use of PHMB for appropriateness to wounds and practicality.

PHMB affects bacteria by inducing structural changes, allowing bactericidal effects to occur. Technological advances have led to PHMB being incorporated into gauze sponges, nonadherent dressings, foam, and biosynthesized cellulose.[54,55] Considerations of PHMB include the required time exposure of the product (from 10 to 15 minutes) for effective antimicrobial effects, thus negating planning on the clinician's part or consideration of use as a continuous irrigant solution. Contradictions to PHMB are previous adverse reactions to PHMB or chlorhexidine as well as the cautious use with any solutions other than normal saline, sterile water, or potable water because of the possibility of yellow staining of the patient.[54,55]

SUMMARY

Patients admitted to critical care units are at high risk for increased morbidity and mortality from skin and deep wound infections. The skin is a complex organ system and the first line of defense against infection. Once breached, a wound is contaminated with natural flora that stimulates the inflammatory process and signals a series of sequential but overlapping phases necessary for wound closure. When a wound cannot progress from the inflammatory phase, delayed healing results and wounds become chronic. Biofilms are a serious problem and difficult to eradicate. It is imperative for clinicians to be more thoughtful in the use of systemic antibiotics because of the continued emergence of multiple drug–resistant bacteria. Antimicrobial therapy should be guided by quantitative culture techniques performed in the correct manner. Numerous commercially available antimicrobial/antiseptic agents have been developed that should be considered as part of a comprehensive wound management strategy.

REFERENCES

1. Sen CK, Gordillo GM, Sashwati R, et al. Human skin wounds: a major and snowballing threat to public health and economy. Wound Repair Regen 2009;17(6): 763–71.
2. Hanberger H, Arman D, Gill H, et al. Surveillance of microbial resistance in European intensive care units: a first report from the Care-ICU program for improved infection control. Intensive Care Med 2009;35:91–100.
3. Pfaller MA, Flamm RK, Sader HS, et al. Ceftaroline activity against bacterial organisms isolated from acute bacterial skin and skin structure infections in the United States medical centers (2009-2011). Diagn Microbiol Infect Dis 2014;78: 422–8.
4. Bordon J, Master RN, Clark RB, et al. Methicillin-resistant *Staphylococcus aureus* to non-β-lactam antimicrobials in the United States from 1996 to 2008. Diagn Microbiol Infect Dis 2010;67:395–8.
5. Sussman C, Bates-Jenson B. Wound care: a collaborative practice manual for health professionals. 4th edition. Baltimore (MD): Lippincott Williams & Wilkins; 2012.
6. Meyers BA. Wound management principles and practice. 2nd edition. Saddle River (NJ): Pearson Prentice Hall; 2008.
7. Baranoski S, Ayello EA. Wound care essentials practice principles. 3rd edition. Philadelphia: Wolters Kluwer Health; 2012.
8. Merad M, Ginhoux F, Collin M. Origin, homeostasis and function of Langerhans cells and other langerin-expressing dendritic cells. Nat Rev Immunol 2008;8: 935–47.
9. Grossman S, Porth CM. Porth's pathophysiology: concepts of altered health states. 9th edition. Philadelphia: Wolters Kluwer Health; 2013.
10. Chen JW, Abatangelo G. Functions of hyaluronan in wound repair. Wound Repair Regen 1999;7(2):79–89.
11. Moore KL, Dalley AF, Agur AMR. Moore clinically oriented anatomy. 7th edition. Philadelphia: Wolters Kluwer Health; 2014.
12. Sibbald RG, Woo K, Ayello EA. Increased bacterial burden and infection: the story of NERDS and STONES. Adv Skin Wound Care 2006;19(8):447–61.
13. Roupe KM, Nybo M, Sjobring U, et al. Injury is a major inducer of epidermal innate immune responses during wound healing. J Invest Dermatol 2010;130: 1167–77.
14. Martin P, Leibovich SJ. Inflammatory cells during wound repair: the good, the bad and the ugly. Trends Cell Biol 2005;15:599–607.
15. Goldberg SR, Diegelmann RF. Wound healing primer. Crit Care Nurs Clin North Am 2012;24(2):165–78.
16. Bryant RA, Nix DP. Acute and chronic wounds: current management concepts. 5th edition. St Louis (MO): Elsevier, Inc; 2016.

17. Landis S, Ryan S, Woo K. Infections in chronic wounds. In: Krasner D, Rodeheaver GT, Sibbald RG, editors. Chronic wound care: a clinical source book for healthcare professional. Malver (PA): HMP Communications; 2007.
18. Wolcott RD, Rhoads DD. A study of biofilm-based wound management subjects with critical limb ischemia. J Wound Care 2008;17(4):145–8.
19. White J, Cutting KF. Critical colonization—the concept under scrutiny. Ostomy Wound Manage 2006;52:52–6.
20. Percival SL, Hill KE, Williams DW, et al. A review of the scientific evidence for biofilms in wounds. Wound Repair Regen 2012;20(5):647–67.
21. James GA, Swogger E, Wolcott R, et al. Biofilms in chronic wounds. Wound Repair Regen 2008;16(1):37–44.
22. Wolcott RD, Rumbaugh KP, James G, et al. Biofilm maturity studies indicated sharp debridement opens a time-dependent therapeutic window. J Wound Care 2010;19(8):320–8.
23. Bradely BH, Cunningham M. Biofilms in chronic wounds and the potential role of negative pressure wound therapy: an integrative review. J Wound Ostomy Continence Nurs 2013;40(2):134–49.
24. Sakarya S, Gunay N, Karakulak M, et al. Hypochlorous acid: an ideal wound care agent with powerful microbicidal, antibiofilm, and wound healing potency. Wounds 2014;26(12):342–50.
25. Edmiston CE, McBain AJ, Roberts C, et al. Clinical and microbiological aspects of biofilm-associated surgical site infections. Adv Exp Med Biol 2015;830:47–67.
26. Malic S, Hill KE, Hayes A, et al. Detection and identification of specific bacteria in wound biofilms using peptide nucleic acid fluorescent in situ hybridization (PNA FISH). Microbiology 2009;155(Pt 8):2603–11.
27. Willey M, Karam M. Impact of infection on fracture fixation. Orthop Clin North Am 2016;47:357–64. Available at: http://dx.doi.org/10.1016/j.ocl.2015.09.004.
28. Dowd SE, Sun Y, Secor PR, et al. Survey of bacterial diversity in chronic wounds using pyrosequencing, DGGW, and full ribosome shotgun sequencing. BMC Microbiol 2008;8:1–43.
29. Sader HS, Farrell DJ, Flamm RK, et al. Antimicrobial susceptibility of gram-negative organisms isolated from patients hospitalized in intensive care units in United States and European hospitals (2009-2011). Diagn Microbiol Infect Dis 2014;78:443–8. Available at: http://dx.doi.org/10.1016/j.diagmicrobio.2013.11.025.
30. Sismaet HJ, Banerjee A, McNish S, et al. Electrochemical detection of *Pseudomonas* in wound exudate samples from patients with chronic wounds. Wound Repair Regen 2016;24(2):366–72.
31. Copeland-Halperin LR, Kaminsky AJ, Bluefeld N, et al. Sample procurement for cultures of infected wounds: a systematic review. J Wound Care 2016;25(Suppl 4):S4–10.
32. Davies CE, Hill KE, Newcombe RG, et al. A prospective study of the microbiology of chronic venous leg ulcers to reevaluate the clinical predictive value of tissue biopsies and swabs. Wound Repair Regen 2007;15(1):17–22.
33. Angel DE, Lloyd P, Carville K, et al. The clinical efficacy of two semi-quantitative wound swabbing techniques in identifying the causative organisms in infected cutaneous wounds. Int Wound J 2011;8(2):176–85.
34. Frankel YM, Melendez JH, Wang NY, et al. Defining wound microbial flora: molecular microbiology opening new horizons. Arch Dermatol 2009;10:1193.
35. Rondas AA, Schols JM, Halfens RJ, et al. Swab versus biopsy for the diagnosis of chronic infected wounds. Adv Skin Wound Care 2013;26(5):211–9.

36. Levine NS, Lindberg RB, Mason AD, et al. The quantitative swab culture and smear: a quick simple method for determining the number of viable aerobic bacteria on open wounds. J Trauma 1976;16(2):89–94.
37. Bonham PA. Swab cultures for diagnosing wound infections: a literature review and clinical guideline. J Wound Ostomy Continence Nurs 2009;36(4):389–95.
38. Ovington LG. Hanging wet-to-dry dressings out to dry. Home Healthc Nurse 2001;19(8):477–83.
39. Bolton LL, Monte K. Moisture and healing: beyond the jargon. Ostomy Wound Manage 2000;46(1A Suppl):51S–62S.
40. Armstrong MH, Price P. Wet-to-dry gauze dressings: fact and fiction. Wounds 2004;16(2):109–13.
41. National Pressure Ulcer Advisory Panel (NPUAP) and European Pressure Ulcer Advisory Panel (EPUAP). Prevention and treatment of pressure ulcers. Washington, DC: NPUAP and EPUAP; 2014.
42. Woo K, Keast D, Parsons N, et al. The cost of wound debridement: a Canadian perspective. Int Wound J 2015;12(4):402–7.
43. Waycaster C, Milne CT. Clinical and economic benefit of enzymatic debridement of pressure ulcers compared to autolytic debridement with a hydrogel dressing. J Med Econ 2013;16(7):976–86.
44. Jovanic A, Ermis R, Mewaldt R, et al. The influence of metal salts, surfactants, and wound care products on the enzymatic activity of collagenase, the wound debriding enzyme. Wounds 2012;24(9):242–53.
45. Zarachi K, Gergor J. The efficacy of maggot debridement therapy–a review of comparative clinical trials. Int Wound J 2012;9(5):469–77.
46. Gray M. Is larval (maggot) debridement effective for removal of necrotic tissue from chronic wounds? J Wound Ostomy Continence Nurs 2008;35(4):378.
47. Konig M, Vanscheidt W, Augustin M, et al. Enzymatic versus autolytic debridement of chronic leg ulcers: a prospective randomized trial. J Wound Care 2005;14(7):320–3.
48. Fernandez R, Griffiths R. Water for wound cleansing. Cochrane Database Syst Rev 2012;(2):CD003861.
49. Moore ZE, Cowman S. Wound cleansing for pressure ulcers. Cochrane Database Syst Rev 2013;(3). CD004983. Available at: http://www.woundsresearch.com/article/evidence-corner-wound-cleansing-how-far-have-we-come#sthash.xngnPPV5.dpuf.
50. Weiss EA, Oldham G, Lin M, et al. Water is a safe and effective alternative to sterile normal saline for wound irrigation prior to suturing: a prospective, double-blind, randomized, controlled clinical trial. BMJ Open 2013;3(1). http://dx.doi.org/10.1136/bmjopen-2012-001504.
51. Angeras MH, Brandberg A, Falk A, et al. Comparison between sterile saline and tap water for the cleaning of acute traumatic soft tissue wounds. Eur J Surg 1992;158(6–7):374–450.
52. McGuinness W, Vella E, Harrison D, et al. Influence of dressing changes on wound temperature. J Wound Care 2004;13(9):383–5.
53. Melling AC, Ali B, Scott EM, et al. Effects of preoperative warming on the incidence of wound infection after clean surgery: a randomized controlled trial. Lancet 2001;358:876–80.
54. Schultz G, Sibbald G, Falanga V, et al. Wound bed preparation: a systematic approach to wound management. Wound Repair Regen 2003;11:1–28.
55. Weir D, Brindel T. Wound dressings. In: Hamm R, editor. Text and atlas of wound diagnosis and treatment. Burr Ridge (IL): McGraw Hill; 2015. p. e001504.

56. Mohammadi AA, Seyed SM, Kiasat M, et al. Efficacy of debridement and wound cleansing with 2% hydrogen peroxide on graft take in the chronic-colonized burn wounds: a randomized controlled clinical trial. Burns 2013;39(6):1131–6.
57. Liden BA. Pearls for practice: hypochlorous acid: its multiple uses for wound care. Ostomy Wound Care 2013;59(9):1–6.
58. Robson MC. Treating chronic wounds with hypochlorous acid disrupts biofilm. Today's Wound Clinic 2014;8(9):1–2.
59. Wang L, Bassiri M, Najafi R, et al. Hypochlorous acid as a potential wound care agent. J Burns Wounds 2007;6:65–79.
60. World Union of Wound Healing Societies (WUWHS). Principles of best practice: wound exudate and the role of dressings. A consensus document. London: MEP Ltd; 2007.
61. O'Neill MA, Vine GJ, Beezer AE, et al. Antimicrobial properties of silver-containing wound dressings: a microcalorimetric study. Int J Pharm 2003;263(1–2):61–8.
62. Sibbald RG, Browne AC, Coutts P, et al. Screening evaluation of an ionized nanocrystalline silver dressing in chronic wound care. Ostomy Wound Manage 2001; 47(10):38–43.
63. Pieper B. Honey-based dressings and wound care. J Wound Ostomy Continence Nurs 2009;36(1):60–6.
64. Asamoah B, Ochieng B, Meetoo D. The clinical role of honey in treating diabetic foot ulcers: a review. Diabetic Foot J 2014;17(1):25–8.
65. Sibbald RG, Ovington LG, Ayello EA, et al. Wound bed preparation 2014 update: management of critical colonization with a gentian violet and methylene blue absorbent antibacterial dressing and elevated levels of matrix metalloproteases with an ovine collagen extracellular matrix dressing. Adv Skin Wound Care 2014;27:1–6.

Infections in the Intensive Care Unit

Posttransplant Infections

Fiona Winterbottom, DNP, MSN, APRN, ACNS-BC, CCRN*,
Misty Jenkins, MSN, APRN, ACNP-BC, CCRN

KEYWORDS

- Posttransplant infections • Posttransplant ICU care • Solid organ transplantation
- Risk factors

KEY POINTS

- Solid organ transplant (SOT) has become a well-established standard of care for end-organ failure.
- The nurse in the intensive care unit may be exposed to these patients at any stage in the care continuum of pretransplant or posttransplant care.
- Factors affecting the incidence of infection after SOT include the type of organ transplanted, anatomic region of transplant, incidence of surgical complications, level of immunosuppression, and antirejection therapy.
- Knowledge of risk factors, timing, and treatments for infections may help to enhance clinical practices and optimize patient safety and clinical outcomes.

INTRODUCTION

Each year in the United States organ transplantation offers a lifeline to more than 25,000 individuals who have end-stage organ dysfunction.[1] The United Network for Organ Sharing keeps a tally of the number of transplant donors and patients waiting for solid organ transplant (SOT). In April 2016, there were more than 120,000 waiting list candidates and just over 1000 donors.[2] According to the United Network for Organ Sharing website, solid organs in most demand are kidneys, with more than 100,000 patients on the waiting list, closely followed by almost 15,000 people waiting for livers.[2] There are approximately 4000 candidates waiting for a heart transplant and a little over 1000 candidates waiting for lung and pancreas transplants.[2] The number of donors for kidney and liver transplantation has increased over the past 5 years,

No conflict of interest.
Pulmonary Critical Care, Ochsner Medical Center, Jefferson Highway, New Orleans, LA 70121, USA
* Corresponding author.
E-mail address: Fwinterbottom@ochsner.org

possibly owing to increased living donor transplants. Five-year survival rates for kidney transplant recipients are roughly 75% and for liver transplant recipients it is around 70%.[3] Transplant recipients are at risk of complications related to surgical procedures, immunosuppressive therapy, and infection.[4] Infection remains the most common complication after SOT.[1,4,5] This article discusses infections in SOT recipients including those with kidney, heart, lungs, and pancreas transplants.

RISK OF INFECTIONS IN SOLID ORGAN TRANSPLANTATION

Early postoperative infection is an important source of morbidity and mortality in SOT recipients. Factors affecting the incidence of infection after SOT include the type of organ transplanted, anatomic region of transplant, incidence of surgical complications, level of immunosuppression, and antirejection therapy.[4] Limited high-level evidence exists about the epidemiology and risk factors for early nosocomial infections in SOT recipients; however, the third edition of the American Society of Transplantation Guidelines for the Prevention and Treatment of Infectious Complications of Solid Organ Transplantation offers a guide for clinical practice by providing evidence where it exists and clinical consensus where critically appraised evidence is limited.[4]

Many of the classic clinical markers and inflammatory signs and symptoms associated with infection are diminished in SOT recipients owing to immunosuppression; therefore, usual indicators such as fever, leukocytosis, and wound erythema are not always appreciated.[3] Additionally, usual pain pathways may be disrupted owing to altered anatomy and organ denervation affecting recognition of infection, and subsequently delaying diagnosis and increasing the risk of morbidity and mortality.[3] Transplant recipients are particularly susceptible to infection during episodes of increased immunosuppression and should be observed closely for signs of infection.[3] Traditional testing methods to seek infectious sources may be limited in the diagnosis of acute disease after transplant because bacterial and fungal cultures often have lower yields and radiographs are often insufficient for diagnosing infections.[3]

PRETRANSPLANT SCREENING

Thorough pretransplant screening is performed to identify infectious diseases that may preclude donor or recipient transplantation. This includes a detailed medical history of prior infections, past travel, place of residence, and exposure to animal and environmental pathogens.[5] Standard screening includes human immunodeficiency virus (HIV), cytomegalovirus (CMV) immunoglobulin (Ig)G antibody, hepatitis B virus (HBV), hepatitis C virus (HCV), rapid plasma reagin, toxoplasma antibody, Epstein-Barr virus antibody, and varicella-zoster virus antibody, with additional testing based on patient history.[5] Chest radiography and microbiologic testing of blood and urine are commonly included in screening processes.[6,7] The donor screening process is influenced by the time sensitive nature of organ transplantation and ability to conduct rapid cycle testing.[6] Organ transplant risk factors can be separated into pretransplant, intraoperative, and posttransplant. The pretransplant risk factors are further divided into donor or recipient.

PRETRANSPLANT RISK FACTORS

A rigorous selection process by a team of highly trained specialists is needed to screen candidates for transplant.[8] Patient risk factors should be assessed including pretransplant infection (especially multidrug resistant [MDR] organisms), severity of illness, functional capacity, psychosocial assessment, and ability for self-care posttransplant.[8,9] Donor-derived infection occurs in approximately 0.2% of deceased donor transplants, but may be mitigated by careful medical and social history, physical assessment of organs, and screening for infection.[10] Transmission of bacteria from MDR bacteria, such as methicillin-resistant *Staphylococcus aureus* (MRSA) and vancomycin-resistant *Enterococcus* (VRE) can result in graft loss and increased morbidity and mortality.[10] Donors with bacteremia may be used; however, it is recommended that these donors receive targeted antimicrobial therapy for at least 1 to 2 days before transplantation and demonstrate clinical improvement.[10] Recipients receiving organs from infected donors should receive a 7- to 10-day course of antibiotics targeted to the organism isolated from the donor.[10]

Donor-derived infections are a result of organ transplants with active and latent infections that may or may not be expected.[10] Examples of infections that are expected in transmission include CMV and HBV whereas, pathogens that may be unexpected include HIV, Chagas, HCV, lymphocytic choriomeningitis virus, *Mycobacterium tuberculosis*, MDR, rabies, and West Nile virus.[10] Additionally, there are group of infections such as West Nile virus, HIV, rabies, lymphocytic choriomeningitis viral infection, and Chagas' disease that are associated with deceased donors.

Some pathogens may not be detected in pretransplant screening owing to delays in seroconversion or sensitivity of testing; therefore, transplantation of organs from deceased donors with fever and viral syndromes may be controversial.[6] Colonization of bacterial and fungal infections in donors presents further infectious concerns for the transplant organ recipients; hence, early recognition along with prophylaxis or treatment of the subclinical infection is recommended.[4] The United States Organ Procurement and Transplantation Network monitors disease transmission through a national registry.[10,11]

INTRAOPERATIVE RISK FACTORS

Multiple factors impact the transplant recipient's risk for infection during the operative period, such as the type of surgical reconstruction, unexpected surgical events, ischemic injury, prolonged operative times, operative field contamination, excessive bleeding, and organ injury.[10] Examples of surgical risks include selection of biliary anastomosis in liver transplant patients leading to postoperative biliary complications and deceased donor dysfunctional kidney allografts that lead to higher rates of urinary tract infection (UTI).[3]

POSTOPERATIVE RISK FACTORS

Posttransplant immunosuppression to prevent rejection is a significant risk factor for opportunistic infections.[4,12-14] Microbiological surveillance and assays that measure immunity to assess infectious risk should be in place for common posttransplant pathogens and MDR bacteria, viruses, and fungi.[4,8] Close attention to transplanted organs is essential to detect complications in vascular supply and organ function that could lead to increased risk for infection and expeditious removal of devices to prevent catheter-related infections is highly recommended.[4]

INFECTION PREVENTION

General preventative strategies include vaccination, universal prophylaxis, and preemptive therapy.[3,6] Ideally, vaccinations should be provided before transplantation because immunosuppression and critical illness may decrease vaccination effectiveness.[3,8] The best time for a vaccination panel that includes live vaccinations and attenuated vaccines is early in the course of the disease and before transplant.[8] Small-pox, oral polio, and Calmette-Guerin's bacillus, and live attenuated vaccinations are contraindicated after transplantation.[8] Lifestyle changes are important after transplantation, and include measures to decrease risk for infection such as hand washing after food preparation, gardening, and contact with feces or secretions.[6] Attention to food preparation, including undercooked meats, unwashed fruits and vegetables, unpasteurized dairy products, and avoiding well water are important for transplant recipients to prevent infections.[5–7]

TIMING OF INFECTIONS AFTER SOLID ORGAN TRANSPLANTATION

Timing of infections after SOT is fairly predictable irrespective of organ type. The 3 common time frames related to SOT can be categorized as early, intermediate, and late (**Table 1**).[3,7] The early time period is within the first month after transplant and is usually associated with bacterial and candidal infections; the intermediate phase relates to months 2 to 6 with infections commonly linked with transplantation; and the late period, after 6 months, comprises infections usually related to chronic rejection.[3,7] Advances in powerful immunosuppressive agents have decreased the incidence of rejection of transplanted organs, but has increased patients' susceptibility to opportunistic infections and cancer.[3,7] Routine antimicrobial prophylaxis for *Pneumocystis jirovecii* and CMV has changed patterns of posttransplant opportunistic infections and influenced emergence of new clinical syndromes, such as polyomavirus type BK nephropathy and other organisms with antimicrobial resistance.[6,15]

Infection in immunosuppressed SOT recipients is often difficult to distinguish because signs and symptoms of infection are often diminished and noninfectious causes of fever, allograft rejection, and toxic drug interactions may exist.[3] In these cases, laboratory testing including quantitative assays can sometimes assist in detection of specific infections.[3,4,16] HBV is an example of an infection transmitted through transplant, where risk can be mitigated through testing transplant candidates for HBV (hepatitis B surface antigen, anti-hepatitis B surface, and anti-hepatitis B core), vaccination, and antiviral prophylaxis.[17]

EARLY POSTTRANSPLANT INFECTIONS (LESS THAN 1 MONTH)

Infections during the early posttransplant period are largely donor derived, recipient derived/colonizers, nosocomial pathogens, or related to complications of surgery such as bacteria and yeast.[3,4,7] At least 50% of bacterial infections after transplantation arise during this early period with many labeled as surgical site infections (SSI) that derive from anastomotic stenosis, leaks, or other surgical complications.[4,7] Fluid collections, devitalized tissues, graft injury, and anastomotic issues are risk factors for development of serious invasive infections.[4,7] Donor-derived bacterial and fungal infections transferred with the allograft should be reported to organ procurement agencies to mitigate risk to other organ recipients and to assess antimicrobial susceptibility, prophylaxis, and need for specimen biopsy.[4,7] Concerns during this period warranting investigation include *Clostridium difficile* colitis, hepatitis, pneumonitis, encephalitis, rash, and leukopenia.[13,14,18]

INTERMEDIATE POSTTRANSPLANT INFECTIONS (1 TO 6 MONTHS)

Infections commonly seen during the intermediate period are opportunistic pathogens in the immunocompromised host. Infections often linked with transplantation are latent pathogens transmitted from donor organs, reactivated within the recipient, or transferred in blood products. Potential pathogens include polyomavirus BK, adenovirus, recurrent HCV, and herpesvirus infections, varicella zoster, CMV, Epstein-Barr virus, lymphoproliferative disorders (posttransplant lymphoproliferative disorder), *P jirovecii* pneumonia, toxoplasmosis, aspergillus, tuberculosis, cryptococcus, *Trypanosoma cruzi*, and *Strongyloides*, which may occur in the absence of appropriate prophylaxis or preventative measures.[4,7] Antibacterial prophylaxis with trimethoprim–sulfamethoxazole is usually administered for UTIs and opportunistic infections such as pneumocystis pneumonia, *Listeria monocytogenes* infection, *Toxoplasma gondii* infection, and infection with sulfa-susceptible *Nocardia* spp.[3,6,7]

LATE POSTTRANSPLANT INFECTIONS (GREATER THAN 6 MONTHS)

The risk of infection usually decreases in the late posttransplant period because immunosuppressive therapy is usually tapered down and allograft function is optimized.[4,7] Individuals who have comorbid conditions such as diabetes mellitus, underlying disease, or malignancy continue to be at an increased risk for infections during this later phase.[4,7] Individuals who require increased immunosuppression, either related to rejection or underlying disease, will be at greater risk for late opportunistic infections.[4,7] Allograft injury can persist owing to chronic viral infections, such as cirrhosis from HCV in liver transplant recipients; *Stenotrophomonas*, *Pseudomonas*, *Aspergillus*, and bronchiolitis obliterans in lung transplant recipients; accelerated vasculopathy in heart-transplant recipients with CMV; and other malignant disorders such as posttransplantation lymphoproliferative disorder.[4,7]

Immunosuppressed transplant patients continue to be at increased risk for opportunistic infection with *listeria* or *Nocardia* spp, invasive fungal pathogens such as zygomycetes and dematiaceous molds, and unusual organisms (eg, *rhodococcus* spp).[4,7]

TYPES OF POSTTRANSPLANT INFECTIONS
Pneumonia

Pneumonia is the most commonly diagnosed nosocomial infection in surgical patients and often is seen in the early phase after SOT as a hospital-acquired pneumonia. These hospital-acquired infections occur after 48 hours of hospital stay with increased risk for patients requiring mechanical ventilation via endotracheal intubation.[1]

Urinary Tract Infection

Diagnosis of UTI in adults requires the presence of dysuria, increased urinary frequency, or suprapubic tenderness, combined with a positive urine culture.[1] The most common causative pathogens are gram-negative bacteria, including *Escherichia coli*, *E cloacae*, and *Acinetobacter baumannii*. High percentages of SOT patients are found to be colonized with MRSA or VRE, leading to increased risk of ensuing infections.[14]

Surgical Site Infection

SSIs are defined as postoperative infections around the surgical incision that are superficial, deep, or have organ involvement and occur within 30 to 90 days after device implantation.[1] Diagnosis of an SSI requires a positive culture from the surgical site, a purulent exudate from a surgical wound, or a surgical incision that requires reopening.[1] SSIs in the general surgical population are considered to be preventable with increased risk among those with advanced age, diabetes, smoking history, obesity, and lengthy operative times.[1] SSIs are linked with longer durations of stay in the

Table 1
Timing of posttransplant infections

Infection type	Early 0–1 mo	Intermediate 1–6 mo	Late >6 mo
Bacterial			
Catheter-related infections, wound infection, pneumonia			
	Gram-negative enteric bacilli Small bowel, liver, neonatal heart *Pseudomonas/Burkholderia* spp. CF: lung Gram-positive MRSA/VRE Anastomotic leaks and ischemia *Clostridium difficile* colitis	*Nocardia* Listeria, *Mycobacterium tuberculosis* Pneumonia CF: lung Gram-negative enteric bacilli *Pseudomonas/Burkholderia* spp. PCP and antiviral (CMV, HBV) prophylaxis: polyomavirus BK infection, nephropathy Small bowel *C difficile* colitis	Community-acquired pneumonia, urinary tract infection *Pseudomonas/ Burkholderia* spp. CF: lung Lung recipients with chronic rejection gram-negative bacillary bacteremia Small bowel Infection with *Nocardia, Rhodococcus* spp.
Viral	Varicella zoster virus *Pseudomonas/ Burkholderia* spp.	*Cryptoccocus neoformans* infection *Mycobacterium tuberculosis* infection Anastomotic complications	CMV retinitis or colitis Papillomavirus, Community-acquired (SARS, West Nile virus infection) JC polyomavirus infection Skin cancer, lymphoma Posttransplant lymphoproliferative disorder HSV encephalitis
	HSV CMV, Epstein–Barr virus, varicella–zoster virus, influenza, posttransplant lymphoproliferative disorder (respiratory syncytial virus), Adenovirus Hepatitis (HBV, HCV)		

| Fungal | Candida spp (non-albicans) | Pneumocystis Aspergillus | Cryptococcus Aspergillus spp. • Lung transplants with chronic rejection Infection with Aspergillus, atypical molds, Mucor spp. |
| Parasitic | | Strongyloides Toxoplasma Leishmania Toxoplasma gondii Trypanosoma cruzi | |

Abbreviations: CF, cystic fibrosis; CMV, cytomegalovirus; HBV, hepatitis B virus; HCV, hepatitis C virus; HSV, herpes simplex virus; MRSA, methicillin-resistant *Staphylococcus aureus*; PCP, *Pneumocystis jirovecii* pneumonia; SARS, severe acute respiratory syndrome; VRE, vancomycin-resistant *Enterococcus*.

intensive care unit (ICU), more frequent hospital readmissions, increased morbidity and mortality, and cost in excess of $40,000 per infected patient.[1]

Blood Stream Infections

Blood stream infections (BSIs) in both the general surgical population and in transplant recipients have been associated with significant morbidity and mortality with increased risks such as red blood cell transfusion, parenteral nutrition, age, immunosuppression, and medical comorbidities, including diabetes, peripheral vascular disease, congestive heart failure, and renal and liver disease.[1] Incidence of BSI within 30 days of SOT ranges from 7% to 14%. The approximate incidence by organ transplanted is 5% in kidney and pancreas-kidney, and 12% in liver transplants. Gram-positive bacteria are most frequently isolated in transplant recipients, although gram-negatives are more frequent among kidney and liver transplant recipients.[1,4,7] Antibiotic resistance is common, with MDR and hospital-acquired infections becoming a significant risk before and after transplantation.[5,12–14]

INFECTIONS AND TYPE OF TRANSPLANT
Kidney Transplant

UTIs are the most common infections after a kidney transplant, likely owing to anatomic disruption of the urinary tract during surgery, presence of ureteral catheters during the first weeks posttransplant, and preexistent urinary tract abnormalities.[1,15,19] Risk factors for BSI in kidney transplant recipients include ABO incompatibility, previous CMV infection, pretransplant dialysis, acute rejection, urologic disease, presence of a ureteral stent, and high posttransplant serum creatinine levels. Gram-negative bacteria identified as the main pathogens responsible for BSI in this group are E coli, Pseudomonas aeruginosa, Klebsiella spp, Enterobacter spp, and A baumanii. Gram-positive bacteria identified as the main pathogens responsible for BSI in this group are coagulase-negative staphylococci, Enterococcus spp, and S aureus.[1,15,16,19] The incidence of candidemia after renal transplantation is low with most common spp identified as C albicans, C parapsilosis, and C glabrata.[16] Kidney transplant recipients are at significant risk for developing infection by MDR pathogens (VRE, MRSA, extended-spectrum betalactamase–producing Klebsiella pneumoniae, carbapenem-resistant A baumannii, carbapenem-resistant P aeruginosa, and extended-spectrum betalactamase–producing Enterobacter spp).[16]

Pneumonia in the Kidney Transplant Patient

The incidence of early nosocomial pneumonia in the kidney transplant recipient range from around 5% to 15% with most common bacterial pathogens including S aureus, P aeruginosa, Acinetobacter spp, and Haemophilus influenzae. Nosocomial pneumonia in kidney transplant recipients has a mortality of 35%.[1]

Urinary Tract Infection in Kidney Transplantation

The most common infection in kidney transplant recipients is UTI with estimates of subsequent bacteremia in up to 60% of these patients.[1,16] Risk factors for nosocomial UTI include age, female gender, duration of bladder catheterization, use of ureteral stents, delayed graft function, immunosuppression regimen, glomerulonephritis, and simultaneous double renal transplant.[1,19] Renal transplant recipients with UTIs are more likely experience a failed transplanted allograft than recipients who do not develop UTIs; therefore, preventive infection control strategies are essential.[1] Early postoperative UTIs are thought to be largely preventable with early catheter removal and implementation of infection evidence-based infection control practices.[19] The most commonly seen UTIs include *E coli*, *K pneumoniae*, and *enterococcus* spp. UTI treatment includes Trimethoprim-sulfamethoxazole prophylaxis and early urinary catheter removal to reduce risk of UTIs.

Surgical Site Infection in Kidney Transplantation

The incidence of SSIs in kidney transplant patients ranges from 7% to 18% with gram-positive bacteria, staphylococci, and enterococci as the most frequently isolated organisms.[1] Risk factors for SSIs in kidney transplant recipients include pretransplant diabetes mellitus, delayed graft function, a high body mass index, pretransplant glomerulonephritis, acute graft rejection, and need for reoperation early posttransplant; each have been implicated as independent risk factors for the development.[1,20]

Blood Stream Infections in Kidney Transplantation

BSI complicates the early postoperative course of up to 5% of renal transplant recipients, with most cases secondary to a UTI, catheter-related, pneumonia, gastrointestinal, and SSIs.[1,19] Risk factors for early BSIs in kidney transplant recipients include acute rejection, hemodialysis before transplantation, local infections, ureteric stent after transplantation, and being a deceased donor organ recipient. Increased risk of 30-day mortality of kidney transplant recipients who develop a BSI is seen in those with an high Acute Physiology And Chronic Health Evaluation (APACHE) II score, the presence of shock at diagnosis, and respiratory failure.[1,9,19]

Liver Transplant Recipients

BSIs are frequent complications in liver transplant recipients in part owing to the risk of relative immunosuppression of cirrhotic patients before transplantation, and to the prolonged surgical procedure of transplantation.[1,21–24] Risk factors for BSI after liver transplantation include diabetes mellitus, hypoproteinemia, catheterization, preoperative massive effusion or ascites, preoperative *S aureus* carriage, posttransplant hemodialysis, operative blood loss, reoperation, need for mechanical ventilation, and bile duct complications.[1,21,22]

Common organisms found in liver transplant patients include gram-negative bacilli (*E coli*), gram-positive bacteria (*S aureus*), and *Candida*.[1,21,22] Studies show that up to 40% of liver transplant recipients develop at least 1 fungal infection after transplantation with other studies showing increased incidence of infection by MDR gram-negative organisms, such as *Stenotrophomonas maltophilia*, *Ochrobactrum anthropi*, *Pseudomonas* spp, and *A baumanii*. Additionally, pretransplant colonization with VRE and MRSA resulted in a significantly higher risk of infection.[16] These infections have a significant impact on mortality with rates as high as 70%.[1,21,22]

Pneumonia in Liver Transplantation

Pneumonia occurs in 14% to 25% of liver transplant recipients with Enterobacteriaceae, *H influenzae*, *P aeruginosa*, and Aspergillus found as the most common causing pathogens.[1,21,22] Risk factors for pneumonia in liver transplant recipients include retransplantation, surgical technique, dialysis, increased international normalized ratio (>2.3) before liver transplantation, restrictive lung physiology, and prolonged mechanical ventilation.[1,21,22] Nosocomial pneumonia in liver transplant patients has been linked to mortalities as high as 40%.[1]

Urinary Tract Infection in Liver Transplantation

Seven percent to 14% of liver transplant recipients experience a symptomatic UTI in the first month after transplantation owing to gram-negative bacteria including *E coli, E cloacae*, and *A baumannii*.[1] Many organisms are MDR organisms that result in suboptimal patient outcomes and increased health care costs (**Table 2**).[20]

Surgical Site Infections in Liver Transplantation

Liver transplantation is a complex procedure that has one of the highest rates of SSIs.[1,21,22] Independent risk factors for SSI in patients undergoing liver resection include preoperative open wound, surgical technique, hypernatremia, hypoalbuminemia, increased serum bilirubin, dialysis, and longer operative time.[1,21,22] Pathogens that cause SSI in adult liver transplant recipients include *Enterococcus* spp, *Staphylococcus* spp, *Candida* spp, and gram-negative bacteria.[1,21,22] SSIs may be identified by induration, erythema, tenderness, or drainage from the incision site.[1] Risk factors for SSIs in liver transplant recipients include increased operative time (>3.5 hours), surgery lasting more than 7 hours, antibiotic therapy within 3 months before liver transplantation, leak at the biliary anastomosis, female gender, HLA mismatches, increased preoperative white blood cell count, and a donor liver mass-to-recipient body mass ratio of less than 0.01.[1,21]

Blood Stream Infections in Liver Transplantation

The incidence of BSI in liver transplant recipients ranges from 10% to 40%, with more than 50% of bacteremias occurring within the first month after transplantation.[1,21] The most frequently isolated pathogens include *S aureus* and coagulase-negative staphylococci, extended-spectrum betalactamase–producing *E coli*, MDR *P aeruginosa*, candidemia, and invasive fungal infections with primary infectious sources of intravascular catheters and surgical wounds.[1,8,21,22] Risk factors for BSIs include diabetes mellitus, serum albumin levels of greater than 3.0 mg/dL, retransplantation, high transfusion requirement (≥40 U of cellular blood products), choledochojejunostomy, posttransplant dialysis, colonization with Candida spp before transplantation, and pretransplant use of fluoroquinolone prophylaxis for spontaneous bacterial peritonitis.[1,8,21,22] Because the in-hospital mortality for invasive candidiasis may be as high as 80%, antifungal prophylaxis is recommended for recipients with more than 2 risk factors for candidemia.[1,8,21,22]

Lung Transplant Recipients

The incidence of BSI in lung transplant recipients is approximately 25% and varies between early and late posttransplant time periods and between cystic fibrosis (CF) and non-CF patients.[25–27] Most common infections include *S aureus*, *P aeruginosa*, and *Candida* spp from vascular catheter and pulmonary sources. Gram-negative BSIs are often owing to MDR pathogens including *P aeruginosa*, *Burkholderia cepacia* group, and *K pneumoniae* isolates, whereas most pulmonary infections were owing to resistant gram-negative pathogens.[25–27] Colonization and bacteremia by *B cepacia* group is recognized as an important mortality risk factor for CF lung transplant recipients because it can result in progressive necrotizing pneumonia with persistent bacteremia that is highly resistant.[16]

Pneumonia in Lung Transplantation

The prevalence of pneumonia in lung transplant recipients may be as high as 60% with highest risk of infection occurring in the first month posttransplant and with highest mortality in CF patients[25–27] Risk factors include bilateral lung transplant, lung volume reduction, redo transplantation, and preoperative colonization with gram-negative rods.[25–27] The most frequently isolated organisms after lung transplantation include *P aeruginosa*, *S aureus*, and *Aspergillus* spp. Most CF patients are colonized with *P*

Table 2
Recommendations for multidrug-resistant pathogens in solid organ transplant recipients

	MRSA	VRE	Extended-spectrum betalactamase, ampC, Carbapenemase-producing gram –negative bacilli	Nonfermentative gram-negative bacilli
Routine screening	√	X	X	X
Contact precautions	√	√	√	√-Lung √
Isolation	√	√	X	√
Decolonization	Mupirocin (nasal) Chlorhexidine (bathing)	X	X	X

In an outbreak or period of high prevalence surveillance screening may be necessary *aeruginosa* by the time they are transplanted, with the paranasal sinuses serving as a reservoir for bacteria. Sinus surgery and daily nasal irrigation with saline has been found to reduce recolonization of the allograft, improve survival, and reduce the incidence of posttransplant bronchiolitis obliterans syndrome. *Aspergillus* remains the most common fungal infection in transplant recipients in the late postoperative period, but may be seen in patients admitted to ICU for respiratory failure.[1,25]

Surgical Site Infections in Lung Transplantation

There are few studies about SSIs in lung transplant recipients; however, the incidence is thought to be approximately 5%, occurring as empyema, surgical wound infection, mediastinitis, sternal osteomyelitis, or pericarditis.[25–27] The most commonly found organisms include *S aureus*, *P aeruginosa*, and *Enterococcus faecium*, along with MDR pathogens, frequently MRSA. Risk factors for SSI include ischemic time, number of red blood cell transfusions, female donor, diabetes, and prior cardiothoracic surgery. Hospital duration of stay, mortality at 6 months, and mortality at 1 year are greater in lung transplant recipients with SSIs.[1]

Pneumonia in Heart Transplantation

The incidence of pneumonia in heart transplant recipients can reach as high as 50%, with commonly isolated pathogens including *S aureus*, *P aeruginosa*, *A baumanii* , and *Enterobacter cloacae*.[1,16] Nosocomial pneumonia is often an early infection after heart transplantation and is associated with increased mortality, especially in patients requiring mechanical ventilation.[1,16,28,29]

Surgical Site Infections in Heart Transplantation

The incidence of SSI after heart transplant can be as high as 40%, which is higher than other cardiac surgeries, and linked to increased morbidity and mortality.[1,16] SSI subtypes are superficial and deep and are caused by gram-positive bacteria (MRSA) and fungal spp (*Candida*).[1,16,28] Risk factors for SSI after heart transplant include body mass index of greater than 30 kg/m^2, previous heart surgery, prolonged cardiopulmonary bypass time, previous ventricular assist device implantation, inotropic support, increased age, and immunosuppression regimens that include sirolimus/tacrolimus. Heart transplant recipients who develop deep sternal wound infections, mediastinitis and wound dehiscence have increased in-hospital mortality compared with patients without infection but do have similar 5-year if they survive the initial infection.[1,16,28]

Blood Stream Infections in Heart Transplantation

The incidence of BSI in heart transplant recipients is up to 15%, with most infections being nosocomial. Central venous catheters, surgical wounds, lower respiratory tract infection, and UTI are the most common sources of bacteremia.[1,16,28] The most common organisms seen posttransplant include gram-negative pathogens, including *E coli*, *P aeruginosa*, *K pneumoniae*, *Serratia marcescens*, and gram-positive microorganisms including *S aureus*, MRSA, *Staphylococcus epidermidis*, and *Enterococcus faecalis*.[1,16] Risk factors for BSI include hemodialysis, prolonged ICU duration of stay, previous CMV infection, and preexisting ventricular assist device at the time of transplantation.[1,16]

Pancreas Transplant Recipients

Pancreas and kidney-pancreas transplant recipients are at risk for bacterial infections from surgical complications, including intraabdominal infections, duodenal leaks, recurrent UTIs, wound infections, pulmonary, and catheter related sources. Common infections include *Enterobacteriaciae*, VRE, and *Acinetobacter* spp.[1,16]

SUMMARY

SOT has become a well-established standard of care for end-organ failure and the ICU nurse may be exposed to these patients at any stage in the care continuum of pre-transplant or posttransplant care. Knowledge of risk factors, timing, and treatments for infections may help to enhance clinical practices and optimize patient safety and clinical outcomes.

REFERENCES

1. Dorschner P, McElroy LM, Ison MG. Nosocomial infections within the first month of solid organ transplantation. Transpl Infect Dis 2014;16(2):171–87.
2. United Network for Organ sharing (UNOS). Transplant Trends. Retrieved April 20th 2016. Available at: https://www.transplantpro.org/technology/transplant-trends/#waitlists_by_organ. Accessed March, 2016.
3. Greendyke WG, Pereira MR. Infectious complications and vaccinations in the posttransplant population. Med Clin North Am 2016;100(3):587–98.
4. Green M. Introduction: infections in solid organ transplantation. Am J Transplant 2013;13(s4):3–8.
5. Fischer SA, Lu K. Screening of donor and recipient in solid organ transplantation. Am J Transplant 2013;13(s4):9–21.
6. Fishman JA. Infection in solid-organ transplant recipients. N Engl J Med 2007; 357(25):2601–14.
7. Fishman JA. Infections in immunocompromised hosts and organ transplant recipients: essentials. Liver Transpl 2011;17(S3):S34–7.
8. Fagiuoli S, Colli A, Bruno R, et al. Management of infections pre- and post-liver transplantation: report of an AISF consensus conference. J Hepatol 2014;60(5): 1075–89.
9. Shao M, Wan Q, Xie W, et al. Bloodstream infections among solid organ transplant recipients: epidemiology, microbiology, associated risk factors for morbidity and mortality. Transplant Rev 2014;28(4):176–81.
10. Ison MG, Grossi P. Donor-derived infections in solid organ transplantation. Am J Transplant 2013;13(s4):22–30.
11. US Department of Health and Human Services. Organ Procurement and Transplantation Network. Policies. Retrieved April 20th 2016 https://optn.transplant.hrsa.gov/media/1200/optn_policies.pdf. Accessed March, 2016.
12. Gallagher C, Smith JA. CNS infections in solid organ transplant recipients. Neurology 2016;9(Part 3):1.
13. Van Duin D, Van Delden C. Multidrug-resistant gram-negative bacteria infections in solid organ transplantation. Am J Transplant 2013;13(s4):31–41.
14. Ziakas PD, Pliakos EE, Zervou FN, et al. MRSA and VRE colonization in solid organ transplantation: a meta-analysis of published studies. Am J Transplant 2014; 14(8):1887–94.
15. Gonzalez S, Escobar-Serna DP, Suarez O, et al. BK virus nephropathy in kidney transplantation: an approach proposal and update on risk factors, diagnosis, and treatment. Transplant Proc 2015;47(6):1777–85. Elsevier.
16. Kritikos A, Manuel O. Bloodstream infections after solid-organ transplantation. Virulence 2016;7(3):329–40.

17. Huprikar S, Danziger-Isakov L, Ahn J, et al. Solid organ transplantation from Hepatitis B Virus–Positive donors: consensus guidelines for recipient management. Am J Transplant 2015;15(5):1162–72.
18. Dubberke ER, Burdette SD. Clostridium difficile infections in solid organ transplantation. Am J Transplant 2013;13(s4):42–9.
19. Guler S, Cimen S, Hurton S, et al. Risks and benefits of early catheter removal after renal transplantation. Transplant Proc 2015;47(10):2855–9. Elsevier.
20. Cervera C, Delden C, Gavaldà J, et al. Multidrug-resistant bacteria in solid organ transplant recipients. Clin Microbiol Infect 2014;20(s7):49–73.
21. Hernandez MD, Martin P, Simkins J. Infectious complications after liver transplantation. Gastroenterol Hepatol 2015;11(11):741–53.
22. Neuberger J. An update on liver transplantation: a critical review. J Autoimmun 2016;66:51–9.
23. Mumtaz K, Faisal N, Husain S, et al. Universal prophylaxis or preemptive strategy for cytomegalovirus disease after liver transplantation: a systematic review and Meta-analysis. Am J Transplant 2015;15(2):472–81.
24. Vlad JL, Teodor M, Hrehoreţ D, et al. Blood culture value in patients with severe infections after liver transplantation. Acta Med Transilvanica 2014;19(4).
25. Remund KF, Best M, Egan JJ. Infections relevant to lung transplantation. Proc Am Thorac Soc 2009;6(1):94–100.
26. Fuehner T, Kuehn C, Welte T, et al. ICU care before and after lung transplantation. Chest 2016;150(2):442–50.
27. Clajus C, Blasi F, Welte T, et al. Therapeutic approach to respiratory infections in lung transplantation. Pulm Pharmacol Ther 2015;32:149–54.
28. Moore-Gibbs A, Bither C. Cardiac transplantation: considerations for the intensive care unit nurse. Crit Care Nurs Clin North Am 2015;27(4):565–75.
29. Awad M, Czer LS, De Robertis MA, et al. Adult heart transplantation following ventricular assist device implantation: early and late outcomes. Transplant Proc 2016;48(1):158–66. Elsevier.

Antibiotic Trends Amid Multidrug-Resistant Gram-Negative Infections in Intensive Care Units

Leanne H. Fowler, DNP, MBA, AGACNP-BC, CCRN, CNE*,
Susan Lee, MSN, APRN, FNP-BC

KEYWORDS

- Antibiotic resistance • Multidrug-resistant • Gram-negative bacteria • ICU

KEY POINTS

- Multidrug-resistant (MDR) gram-negative bacteria are emerging as the most common nosocomial infections acquired in ICUs worldwide.
- There are multiple strategies with strong supporting evidence that can be used to combat the emergence of MDR gram-negative bacteria.
- Initially inappropriate antibiotic treatments are the leading cause of the emergence of bacterial resistance as the organisms mutate rapidly to protect themselves.
- *Acinetobacter baumannii* and *Pseudomonas aeruginosa* are the leading pathogens worldwide demonstrating virulence against antibiotics.
- Novel treatments and strategies have been proved effective against the emergence of MDR gram-negative pathogens.

ICU admission is significant risk factor for nosocomial bacterial infections.[1,2] Isolates from ICUs internationally most commonly find MDR gram-negative bacteria.[1–8] Multiple studies indicate the leading factor perpetuating antimicrobial resistance is antibiotic misuse.[9–16] The purpose of this article is to discuss the significant impact MDR gram-negative infections are having on ICUs , the threat on health and mortality, and effective and new approaches aimed to combat MDR gram-negative infections in the critically ill population.

BACKGROUND AND PROBLEM
Mechanisms of Antibiotic Resistance

Bacteria become resistant to antibiotics via gene mutations. Gene mutations of the bacteria can occur in 2 ways, intrinsically or from acquired mutations. Intrinsic

Disclosure Statement: The authors have nothing to disclose.
School of Nursing, Louisiana State University Health Sciences Center, 1900 Gravier Street, New Orleans, LA 70112, USA
* Corresponding author.
E-mail address: lfowle@lsuhsc.edu

mutations occur as a defense mechanism to protect against an antibiotic. Acquired resistant gene mutations occur by the transfer of a gene to neighboring bacteria during plasmid exchange.[1,17]

Bacteria demonstrate antibiotic resistance in 4 ways. Bacteria can express enzymes that inactivate or destroy an antibiotic. For instance, bacteria resistant to penicillin produce lactamase. Lactamase breaks down the structure of penicillin, thereby inhibiting its ability to kill or stagnate a microorganism. Despite pharmaceutical companies developing antibiotics able to combat this resistance with β-lactamase inhibitors (β-lactam antimicrobials), the prevalence of extended-spectrum β-lactamase (ESBL) emerged more in the United States than in the rest of the world. Germs expressing ESBL became resistant to most β-lactams, penicillins, third-generation and fourth-generation cephalosporins, and aztreonam. Unfortunately, as the name suggests, ESBL-producing bacteria continue to mutate and some strains have developed coresistance to trimethoprim-sulfamethoxazole, fluoroquinolones, and aminoglycosides.[1]

A second resistance mechanism affects intracellular accumulation of the medications by modifying the target molecule's drug transporters in the microorganism's membrane.[17] The third mechanism involves mutations at the drug's binding site. This limits the ability of the antibiotic to bind tightly to the organism.[1] The last mechanism by which bacteria demonstrate resistance to antibiotics is down-regulating the outer membrane's porin channels and preventing the antibiotic from entering the microorganism's cell.[1]

Biofilm formation and colonization

Many bacteria are capable of protecting themselves by creating a protective coating around the cell known as a biofilm. This coating protects them from the activity of the antibiotic and facilitates resistance.[5,17–20] The biofilm creates protected colonies of the bacteria that are resistant to host defenses and treatments. *A baumannii* is one of the MDR germs that is capable of creating a biofilm.[18–20] These organisms can seed different areas of the body, such as the lung, and cause infections later when a host's immunity is weakened again.[17]

Epidemiology and Emergence of Gram-Negative Bacterial Resistance in ICUs

The Study for Monitoring Antimicrobial Resistance Trends (SMART) reports a global increase and spread of antimicrobial resistance in bacteria causing hospital-associated and community-associated infections.[2] Specifically in ICUs, isolates of gram-negative bacteria have demonstrated MDR trends worldwide increasingly for more than 10 years.[3,5,8,9,13,21] Patients admitted to ICUs for noninfectious causes are at high risk for MDR nosocomial infections due to contamination of equipment, mechanical ventilation, invasive lines/catheters, contamination of surfaces, and contamination of ICU staff.[4–6] Although an MDR gram-negative infection has not been found a single predictor of mortality, the presence of this infection compounded by ICU admission greater than 48 hours, the presence of invasive lines, and other comorbidities greatly increases the overall ICU mortality rate in comparison with non-MDR gram-negative infection diagnoses.[6]

Sepsis related to intraabdominal or pulmonary sources is a diagnosis associated with the highest ICU mortality rates secondary to MDR gram-negative organisms.[2] Patients who have undergone severe burns of the head and neck region are identified at high risk for MDR gram-negative infections as well.[22] In addition to the already troubling and lethal risks for death, those patients colonized with MDR gram-negative bacteria (eg, nursing home residents, individuals with chronic renal disease, immunocompromised individuals, and those with frequent hospital visits) are at an increased risk for a more virulent and invasive infection as well as higher mortality rate.[18,19,21] The emergence of MDR gram-negative organisms was rising as treatments they were susceptible to were declining.[2,8,11–13] Given the alarming rates of death and high costs of health care associated with MDR gram-negative infections, new developments in adequate treatment and reliable methods to delay and prevent resistance were in great demand.

Cross-contamination
MDR gram-negative organisms' emergence has threatened not only ICUs but also other areas in the hospital. Studies revealed transmission of MDR gram-negative isolates found in ICUs were also found in emergency departments and on lower-acuity units within the hospitals.[4,9,12–14,19,22] Theories hypothesize this transmission is due to staff cross-contaminating different areas of the hospitals via their clothing after caring for patients; patients who are colonized (eg, nursing home patients and bedridden patients) also cross-contaminate different areas in the hospital when transported or transferred to another unit.[4,9,12,14] Fortunately, the use of contact precautions and screening for the colonization of virulent MDR germs have strong evidence supporting these measures in reducing the outbreak.[13,23]

Most Common Multidrug-resistant Gram-Negative Microorganisms in ICUs

A baumannii is arguably the leading MDR opportunistic pathogen emerging within ICUs globally.[1,2,9,11] *P aeruginosa* is another prevalent germ, however, found globally with increasing resistance against multiple antibiotics.[1,2,10,11] It is important for clinicians to know the prevalence of specific germs varies greatly according to geographic regions. Therefore, the use of a facility-specific or region-specific antibiogram and expertise of an infectious diseases specialist are vital to the appropriate treatment and reduction of the resistance of these pathogens.[1]

There are many acronyms used to remember the most common MDR gram-negative germs. SPACE organisms identify a group of highly resistant germs to β-lactam antibiotics and consist of *Serratia marcescens, Pseudomonas aeruginosa, Acinetobacter* species, *Citrobacter* species, and *Enterobacter* species,[1] whereas ESKAPE organisms (*Enterococcus faecium, Staphylococci aureus, Klebsiella pneumoniae, Acinetobacter* species, *P aeruginosa,* and *Enterobacter* species) represent the 6 most common MDR pathogens threatening patients within the ICU environment and include the infamous gram-positive *S aureus*.[10] Acronyms help clinicians remember the most prevalent germs; however, it is more important to know the most prevalent organisms emerging within a geographic region.

CLINICAL MANAGEMENT
Antibiotic Stewardship

As discussed previously, inappropriate or misuse of antibiotics is the leading cause of bacterial resistance. Identifying infectious etiologies of critically ill patients can be challenging, and withholding antibiotic therapy until full manifestation of an infection could contribute to ICU mortality. Researchers persist in attempting to identify markers specific to sepsis or to severe infections contributing to critical illness. In the meantime, medical providers must maintain prudence in measures found to prevent bacterial resistance within the hospital overall but in the ICU especially.[2,11]

The 2016 guidelines of the Infectious Diseases Society of America[24] in collaboration with other national organizations have confirmed maintaining an antibiotic stewardship program (ASP) improves patient outcomes, reduces adverse events, improves rates of antibiotic susceptibilities, and maximizes resource utilization. Antibiotic stewardship is now defined in a consensus statement by these organizations as "coordinated interventions designed to improve and measure the appropriate use of [antibiotic] agents by promoting the selection of the optimal [antibiotic] drug regimen including dosing, duration of therapy, and route of administration." Said programs are best led by infectious disease physicians with a multidisciplinary team including, but not limited to, a clinical pharmacist, an infection control nurse, and microbiologist. The new recommendation for ICU antibiotic monitoring is the use of a procalcitonin level to guide point-of-care decision making for the use of antibiotics. Although the guidelines suggest this recommendation had moderate quality of evidence, it lent an opportunity to ASP teams to determine its best use in their facility. The new ASP guidelines do not directly address MDR; however, facilitating the appropriate use of antibiotics has been proved to reduce the prevalence of bacterial resistance.[13,22–24]

Pharmacokinetics in the Critically Ill

The absorption and metabolism of antibiotics is significantly changed in critically ill patients. Critically ill patients' altered pharmacokinetics is due to alterations in body fluid distribution, which has an impact on protein binding, drug elimination, and plasma concentrations of the antibiotic. An ICU patient's alterations can range from a hyperdynamic state where drug clearance is increased and plasma concentrations are increased to the patient requiring maximal life or organ support where fluid alterations have a negative impact on protein binding due to dependence on artificial waste removal and perfusion processes (eg, renal replacement therapy and extracorporeal membrane oxygenation) and unpredictable plasma concentrations of the antibiotic.[21,23]

Pharmacotherapeutics for Multidrug-resistant Gram-Negative Infections

Appropriate selection

Resistant organisms are most commonly found in patients with prior exposure of antibiotics. Clinicians must identify if an ICU patient has suspicion for infection and, if possible, whether the patient received antibiotics recently (within 3 months), which medications were used, and what kind of infection was treated. Another consideration is the anatomic region of the body where some MDR gram-negative organisms normally colonize and may have different resistance patterns in the urine in comparison to those organisms found in the blood or lungs.[21,23] Last but not least, prescribers must consider a patient's risk factors for attaining an MDR gram-negative organism by identifying if the patient is a nursing home resident, received chemotherapy recently, is immunocompromised, has end-stage chronic kidney disease, or has been admitted to a hospital or ICU recently.[8,12]

Rapid germ identification

Novel approaches to rapid identification are currently being studied to identify the molecular structure of germs for species identification. This approach can benefit patients with MDR gram-negative infections given their virulence and association with high mortality in the critically ill population. More research must be conducted to identify the practicality, cost efficiency, and overall clinical significance of using such tests.[25,26]

Novel drug development

The CDC reported the burden antibiotic-resistant organisms posed on health in the United States in 2013. An action was released with the same report imploring for more surveillance of the emerging resistance patterns and the development of new strategies to improve antibiotic use.[27] In response to the CDC's 2013 report, in 2015 the Obama Administration doubled funding to combat antibiotic resistance.[28] Fortunately, there are a few novel therapies for MDR gram-negative infections plaguing ICUs worldwide.

Monotherapies
The 2015 SMART report suggests good in vitro activity against the most common MDR gram-negative organisms persists with amikacin and ertapenem alone in ICU settings.[2] Carbapenems have traditionally been the drugs of choice for MDR gram-negative infections.[1] Intravenous minocycline is also proved effective alone but only as a last resort and guided by an infectious diseases specialist.[29] Given minocycline's adequacy to treat complicated/MDR infections, restraining its use limits the germ's ability to become resistant to it.[24] A study conducted in Malaysia found an increased biofilm production over *A baumannii* when imipenem was used as treatment alone.[20]

Combination therapies
Combination antibiotic therapies demonstrate the most promise in multiple studies looking for the most effective treatment of MDR *A baumannii* and *P aeruginosa*.[21,22,30] The use of antibiotics once effective as monotherapy is now being combined with others to combat the resistant mutations of gram-negative organisms. For example, the use of colistin and polymyxin B has been found to significantly reduce polymixin resistance and demonstrated marked improvement in effectively killing MDR *A baumannii* strains.[30] Fluoroquinolones and aminoglycosides can be effective but are showing increasing resistance to many gram-negative organisms.[1] Another example of combination therapies includes the use of colistin and rifampicin in successfully treating a nosocomial meningitis growing *A baumannii*.[31] Other combination therapies proved to effectively treat MDR *A baumannii* and/or *P aeruginosa* include vancomycin with colistin,[32] cefoperazone or sulbactam with tanreqing,[21] and different variations of β-lactams with β-lactamase inhibitors.[15]

Novel approach
Researchers question if a vaccine can be useful as alternative treatment of MDR *A baumannii*. Immunization of mice with an inactivated vaccine made from antibiotic-exposed MDR *A baumannii* found a higher bactericidal effect against the germ than in those unvaccinated. With further research to gain stronger evidence, the vaccine may provide some protection against MDR *A baumannii* infections.[33]

Strategies to improve efficacy of treatment
Given the demand is high for effective treatments of MDR gram-negative infections, yet the supply of effective treatments is limited, there are multiple approaches to reduce the emergence of MDR organisms in hospitals and ICUs. In addition to maintaining ASPs, researchers are studying the utility of checking therapeutic drug levels for more patients in ICU in consideration of the alterations in pharmacokinetics of antibiotics in the critically ill. Therapeutic drug levels can inform a prescriber when plasma concentrations are too high or too low. As discussed previously, studies show utility in using procalcitonin levels to guide decision making for antibiotic duration.[10] Dose optimization strategies applied to β-lactams, quinolones, and vancomycin administration have shown effectiveness in treating MDR gram-negative bacteria by overcoming the minimum inhibitory concentration and resistance with maintaining high serum concentrations of the antibiotic.[1] These antibiotics achieve optimal bacteria kill rates when serum concentration of the drug is maintained 4 to 5 times higher than the minimum inhibitory concentration.[10] This is achieved by increasing the

dose, decreasing the dosing interval, prolonging the infusion time, or continual infusions of the antibiotic.[1,10] There used to be a theory to cycle antibiotic use within facilities to decrease exposure of the drug to germs. The 2016 Infectious Diseases Society of America guidelines, however, no longer support cycling of antibiotics because there was no strong evidence to support its effectiveness.[24]

IMPLICATIONS FOR PRACTICE

Critical care clinicians must be vigilant in identifying infectious causes of illness as early as possible. Staff nurses must adequately communicate findings to medical providers in a collaborative effort to provide early and appropriate treatment. All critical care clinicians must consider those patients at risk for MDR gram-negative infection given its difficulty to treat and association with high mortality rates when accompanying critical illness.

IMPLICATIONS FOR FUTURE RESEARCH

Critically appraised guidelines aid clinicians' point-of-care decisions for antibiotic stewardship. Little is studied or discussed, however, in the best standards of care, specifically for MDR organisms. Future research is needed to direct non–infectious disease specialists on early treatments of patients with MDR infections.

SUMMARY

Critically ill patients with MDR gram-negative infections have limited options for treatment. Using a prudent ASP multidisciplinary team has proved to minimize inappropriate treatments and consequently reduce the persistence of MDR organisms. Early antibiotic treatment should be guided with consideration of the current research for treatment and the risk factors for and complications of MDR gram-negative infections until infectious diseases expertise can be consulted.

REFERENCES

1. Guervil DJ, Chau T. Trends in multidrug-resistant gram-negative bacilli and the role of prolonged b-lactam infusion in the intensive care unit. Crit Care Nurs Q 2013;36:345–55.
2. Hackel MA, Badal RE, Bouchillon SK, et al. Resistance rates of intra-agcominal isolates from intensive care units and non-intensive care units in the United States: the study for monitoring antimicrobial resistance trends 2010-2012. Surg Infect (Larchmt) 2015;16:298–304.
3. Cobos-Trigueros N, Sole M, Torres JL, et al. Acquisition of Pseudomonas aeruginosa and its resistance phenotypes in critically ill medical patients: role of colonization pressure and antibiotic exposure. Crit Care 2015;4:218.
4. Weiss N, Faugeras F, Roaut B, et al. Multidrug-resistant bacteria transmitted through high-density EEG in ICU. Seizure 2016;4:65–8.
5. Duarte A, Ferreira S, Almeida S, et al. Clinical isolates of Acinetobacter baumannii from a portuguese hospital: PFGE characterization, antibiotic susceptibility and biofilm-forming ability. Comp Immunol Microgiol Infect Dis 2016;4:29–33.
6. Mitharwal SM, Yaddanapudi S, Bhardwaj N, et al. Intensive care unit-acquired infections in a tertiary care hospital: an epidemiologic survey and influence on patient outcomes. Am J Infect Control 2016;44:e113–7.

7. Brotfain E, Borer A, Koyfman L, et al. Multidrug resistance Acinetobacter bacter-emia secondary to ventilator-associated pneumonia: risk factors and outcomes. J Intensive Care Med 2016. [Epub ahead of print].
8. Harris AD, Jackson SS, Robinson G, et al. Pseudomonas aeruginosa colonization in the intensive care unit: prevalence, risk factors, and clinical outcomes. Infect Control Hosp Epidemiol 2016;2:1–5.
9. Mohajeri P, Farahani A, Feizabadi MM, et al. Clonal evolution multi-drug resistant acinetobacter baumannii by pulse-field electrophoresis. Indian J Med Microbiol 2015;33:87–91.
10. Sarin K, Vadivelan M, Bammigatti C. Antimicrobial therapy in the intensive care unit. Indian J Clin Pract 2013;23:601–9.
11. Zilberg MD, Shorr AF, Micek ST, et al. Multi-drug resistance, inappropriate initial antibiotic therapy and mortality in gram-negative severe sepsis and septic shock: a retrospective cohort study. Crit Care 2014;18:596.
12. Cerceo E, Deitelzweig SB, Sherman BM, et al. Multidrug-resistant gram-negative bacterial infections in the hospital setting: overview, implications for clinical prac-tice, and emerging treatment options. Microb Drug Resist 2016;22(5):412–31.
13. Cheon S, Kim MJ, Yun SJ, et al. Controlling endemic multidrug-resistant Acineto-bacter baumannii in intensive care units using antimicrobial stewardship and infection control. Korean J Intern Med 2016;31:367–74.
14. Batarseh A, Al-Sarhan A, Maayteh M, et al. Antibiogram of multidrug resistant Acinetobacter baumannii isolated from clinical specimens at King Hussein Med-ical Centre, Jordan: a retrospective analysis. East Mediterr Health J 2016;21:828–34.
15. MacVane SH. Antimicrobial resistance in the intensive care unit: a focus on gram-negative bacterial infections. J Intensive Care Med 2016. [Epub ahead of print].
16. He L, Meng J, Huang D, et al. Multidrug-resistant Acinetobacter baumannii infec-tion in intensive care unit: a retrospective analysis. Zhong Nan Da Xue Xue Bao Yi Xue Ban 2015;40:1327–32.
17. McCance KL, Huether SE, Brashers VL, et al. Pathophysiology: the biologic basis for disease in adults and children. 6th edition. Maryland Heights (MO): Mosby/Elsevier; 2010.
18. Chang D, Garcia RA, Akers KS, et al. Activity of gallium meso- and protoporphy-rin IX against biofilms of multidrug-resistant Acinetobacter baumannii isolates. Pharmaceuticals 2016;17:E16.
19. Green C, Vadlamudi G, Newton D, et al. The influence of biofilm formation and multidrug resistance on environmental survival of clinical and environmental iso-lates of Acinetobacter baumannii. Am J Infect Control 2016;44(5):e65–71.
20. Dhabaan GN, AbuBakar S, Cerqueira GM, et al. Imipenem treatment induces expression of important genes and phenotypes in a resistant Acinetobacter bau-mannii isolate. Antimicrob Agents Chemother 2015;60:1370–6.
21. Pan T, Liu X, Xiang S, et al. Treatment for patients with multidrug resistant acine-tobacter baumannii pulmonary infection. Exp Ther Med 2016;11:1345–7.
22. Sanchez M, Herruzo R, Marban A, et al. Risk factors for outbreaks of multidrug-resistant Klebsiella pneumonia in critical burn patients. J Burn Care Res 2012;33:386–92.
23. Luyt CE, Brechot N, Trouillet JL, et al. Antibiotic stewardship in the intensive care unit. Crit Care 2014;18:480.
24. Barlam TF, Cosgrove SE, Abbo LM, et al. Implementing an antibiotic stewardship program: guidelines by the infectious diseases society of America and the soci-ety for healthcare epidemiology of America. Clin Infect Dis 2016;62:e51.

25. Huang AM, Newton D, Kunapuli A, et al. Impact of rapid organism identification via matrix-assisted laser desorption/ionization time-of-flight combined with antimicrobial stewardship team intervention in adult patients with bacteremia and candidemia. Clin Infect Dis 2013;57:1237–45.

26. Perez KK, Olsen RJ, Musick WL, et al. Integrating rapid pathogen identification and antimicrobial stewardship significantly decreases hospital costs. Arch Pathol Lab Med 2013;137:1247–54.

27. Centers for Disease Control and Prevention [CDC]a. Antibiotic resistance threats in the United States. 2013. Available at: http://www.cdc.gov/drugresistance/pdf/ar-threats-2013-508.pdf. Accessed April 27, 2016.

28. Centers for Disease Control and Prevention [CDC]b. Antibiotic resistance solutions initiative. 2015. Available at: http://www.cdc.gov/drugresistance/solutions-initiative/index.html. Accessed April 27, 2016.

29. Colton B, McConeghy KW, Schreckenberger PC, et al. IV minocycline revisited for infections caused by multidrug-resistant organisms. Am J Health Syst Pharm 2016;73:279–85.

30. Cheah SE, Li J, Tsuji BT, et al. Colistin and polymyxin B dosage regimens against Acinetobacter baumannii: differences in activity and the emergence of resistance. Antimicrob Agents Chemother 2016;60(7):3921–33.

31. Souhail D, Bouchra B, Belarj B, et al. Place of colistin-rifampicin association in the treatment of multidrug-resistant Acinetobacter baumannii meningitis: a case study. Case Rep Infect Dis 2016;2016:8794696.

32. Yang H, Lv N, Hu L, et al. In vivo activity of vancomycin combined with colistin against multidrug resistant strains of A. baumannii in a Gallleria mellonella model. Infect Dis (Lond) 2016;48:189–94.

33. Shu MH, MatRahim N, NorAmdan N, et al. An inactivated antibiotic-exposed whole-cell vaccine enhances bactericidal activites against multidrug-resistant acinetobacter baumannii. Sci Rep 2016;29:223–32.

Interpreting Laboratory Tests in Infection

Making Sense of Biomarkers in Sepsis and Systemic Inflammatory Response Syndrome for Intensive Care Unit Patients

Jennifer B. Martin, DNP, CRNA, APRN*,
Jennifer E. Badeaux, DNP, CRNA, APRN

KEYWORDS

• Biomarkers • Sepsis • Infection • Inflammation • SIRS • Intensive care

KEY POINTS

- Sepsis and severe sepsis are leading causes of death in the United States and the most common causes of death among critically ill patients in noncoronary intensive care units.
- Diagnosis of infection and sepsis is a subjective clinical judgment that is not sufficiently specific and is often misleading in intensively treated patients.
- No biomarkers have sufficient specificity or sensitivity to be routinely used in clinical practice to differentiate infection and inflammation.
- By diagnosing sepsis early and efficiently, patient care and outcomes will improve by identifying those patients in need of acute care, monitoring therapeutic response, restricting antibiotic usage, and allocating resources most appropriately.
- For intensive care unit nurses, a better understanding of biomarkers as an adjunct to recognizing infection versus inflammation may lead to improved patient outcomes.

INTRODUCTION

For intensive care unit (ICU) bedside practitioners, the diagnosis of infection and sepsis versus inflammation is not an objective, straightforward decision. It is ambiguous and subjective because of the presence of the criteria for systemic inflammatory response syndrome (SIRS), which are sensitive but lack specificity. The physiologic signs and symptoms of sepsis, fever, hypotension, and hypoperfusion, are indistinct and can be caused by a variety of other disease states. Traditional laboratory findings

Disclosure: The authors have nothing to disclose.
Nurse Anesthesia Program, School of Nursing, Louisiana State University Health Sciences Center, 1900 Gravier Street, New Orleans, LA 70112, USA
* Corresponding author.
E-mail address: jmar19@lsuhsc.edu

Crit Care Nurs Clin N Am 29 (2017) 119–130
http://dx.doi.org/10.1016/j.cnc.2016.09.004
0899-5885/17/© 2016 Elsevier Inc. All rights reserved.
ccnursing.theclinics.com

and microbiological cultures have been the standard diagnostic measures, along with hemodynamic measurements and patient assessment. However, in the last 10 to 15 years, data have emerged regarding the use of biomarkers as an adjunct in diagnosis and treatment of infection versus inflammation. Researchers have been able to provide bedside ICU health care teams with vital information regarding the integration of biomarkers into their daily patient assessment in order to make real-time decisions regarding medication treatments for ICU patients. Biomarkers must be target specific and sensitive, easy to implement and interpret, and be cost-effective for routine diagnosis and treatment of critically ill patients. This article informs bedside ICU practitioners regarding the use of biomarkers and their importance in differentiating infection versus inflammation. This knowledge is useful for early diagnosis and treatment in critically ill patients.

BACKGROUND
Prevalence and Incidence

Sepsis and severe sepsis are important and alarming public health issues. Sepsis is a systemic, deleterious host response to infection leading to severe sepsis (acute organ dysfunction secondary to documented or suspected infection) and septic shock (severe sepsis plus hypotension not reversed with fluid resuscitation). Sepsis is defined as the presence (probable or documented) of infection together with systemic manifestations of infection. Severe sepsis is defined as sepsis plus sepsis-induced organ dysfunction or tissue hypoperfusion.[1]

In the United States, sepsis and severe sepsis continue to be the leading causes of death and the most common cause of death among critically ill patients in noncoronary ICUs.[2] The hospitalization rate caused by sepsis as a principal diagnosis has increased more than 2-fold, from 11.6 to 24.0 per 10,000 population between 2001 and 2008.[3] Sepsis accounts for more than 751,000 cases and 215,000 deaths in the United States annually.[2] The incidence of severe sepsis is estimated to be 300 cases per 100,000 people in the United States population, with approximately half of these cases occurring outside of an ICU setting.[2] Data reported recently suggest an annual cost of $14 billion to $16 billion for hospital care of patients with septicemia.[2,4] Respiratory tract infections, especially pneumonia, are the most common site of infection. These types of infection are also associated with the highest mortalities.[5]

Clinical Significance

ICU practitioners are faced with a daily quandary of deciding whether the patient has a new-onset infection versus a persisting inflammatory process. Bedside ICU nurses, along with other members of the interdisciplinary health care team, must collaborate and determine whether a new course of antimicrobials is warranted versus waiting and observing the patient's physical condition. Traditional laboratory findings, along with patient assessment, have been the standard in diagnostic measures until recently. Biomarkers have emerged as useful and effective tools as adjuncts to the traditional diagnostic measures of determining whether a patient is dealing with sepsis or an inflammatory response such as SIRS. However, to date no ideal biomarker has been identified to accomplish this task.

PATHOPHYSIOLOGY

Sepsis and severe sepsis can result from a primary blood infection or from an infection occurring in any part of the body. In patients with systemic infections, the physiologic response can be staged on a continuum from an SIRS, to sepsis, severe sepsis, and septic shock. Septic shock is a type of distributive shock that can also be associated with inflammation of the pancreas and liver, burns, multiple traumatic injuries, anaphylaxis/anaphylactoid reactions, drug or toxin reactions, and transfusion reactions.[2] Each disease process is described here with definitions (**Table 1**).

Systemic Inflammatory Response Syndrome

SIRS is a syndrome that is the consequence of a deregulated inflammatory response to an infectious or noninfectious insult. SIRS, sepsis, severe sepsis, and septic shock were initially defined in 1991 by a consensus panel convened by the American College of Chest Physicians and Society of Critical Care Medicine (American College of Chest Physicians/Society of Critical Care Medicine Consensus Conference).[9]

The term SIRS has routinely been associated with both infectious processes (sepsis) and noninfectious insults, such as an autoimmune disorder, pancreatitis, vasculitis, thromboembolism, burns, or surgery. SIRS was previously defined as 2 or more abnormalities in temperature, heart rate, respiration, or white blood cell count.[6]

Table 1
Definitions of common terms

Condition	Definition/Criteria
SIRS	Syndrome that is the consequence of a deregulated inflammatory response to an infectious or noninfectious insult.[6] Two or more of the following must be present[6]: • Temperature >38°C or <36°C • Heart rate >90 beats/min • Respiratory rate >20/min or $Paco_2$ <32 mmHg (4.3 kPa) White blood cell count >12,000/mm^3 or <4000/mm^3 or >10% immature bands
Sepsis	Complex syndrome resulting from the innate host response to invasive infection[8]
Severe sepsis	Severe sepsis refers to sepsis-induced tissue hypoperfusion or organ dysfunction with any of the following thought to be caused by the infection[6]: • Sepsis-induced hypotension • Lactate level above upper limits of laboratory normal (>0.5–1.6 mmol/L) • Urine output <0.5 mL/kg/h for more than 2 h despite adequate fluid resuscitation • Acute lung injury with Pao_2/Fio_2 <250 mmHg in the absence of pneumonia as infection source • Acute lung injury with Pao_2/Fio_2 <200 mmHg in the presence of pneumonia as infection source • Creatinine level >2 mg/dL (176.8 μmol/L) • Bilirubin level >4 mg/dL (70 μmol/L) • Platelet count <100,000 μL^{-1} • Coagulopathy (INR >1.5)
Septic shock	Septic shock is defined as sepsis-induced hypotension persisting despite adequate fluid resuscitation, which may be defined as infusion of 30 mL/kg of crystalloids (a portion of this may be albumin equivalent). Septic shock is a type of vasodilatory or distributive shock. It results from a marked reduction in systemic vascular resistance, often associated with an increase in cardiac output[7]

Abbreviations: Fio_2, fraction of inspired oxygen; INR, International Normalized Ratio.

Sepsis

Sepsis is defined as the presence (probable or documented) of infection together with systemic manifestations, including fever or hypothermia, tachycardia, and tachypnea.[6] It is assessed by patient presentation, abnormal laboratory findings, physical assessment, and hemodynamic variables. Sepsis management requires a multidisciplinary team of physicians, nurses, pharmacists, respiratory therapists, and nutritionists to maximize the success of therapy for the ICU patient.[7]

Severe Sepsis

Severe sepsis is defined as sepsis-induced organ dysfunction or tissue hypoperfusion, in addition to the diagnosis of sepsis. It is characterized by oliguria, increased creatinine and bilirubin levels, platelet count less than 100,000/μL, and coagulopathy.[7]

Sepsis-induced hypotension, in the absence of other causes of hypotension, is defined as:

1. A systolic blood pressure (SBP) less than 90 mmHg or
2. A mean arterial pressure (MAP) less than 70 mmHg or
3. An SBP decrease greater than 40 mmHg or less than 2 standard deviations below normal for age.[7]

Septic Shock

Septic shock is defined as "sepsis-induced hypotension persisting despite adequate fluid resuscitation."[7] The term sepsis-induced hypoperfusion is defined as hypotension resulting from infection, an increased lactate level, or oliguria.[7] Septic shock is the result of the cascade of inflammation and coagulation, cardiovascular insufficiency, and multiple organ failure. These processes, in combination, often lead to death.[3] However, in practice, the clinical definition and pathophysiology are equivocal such that SIRS and early sepsis cannot be readily distinguished (**Fig. 1**). Thus, when SIRS is suspected it should prompt an evaluation for a septic focus.

DIAGNOSTIC MEASURES
Patient Presentation

Diagnosing sepsis can be difficult because of the variability of signs and symptoms depending on the nature, source, and stage of the infection. A typical patient presentation includes fever or hypothermia, increased white blood cell count, and tachycardia, which can also be caused by a variety of other conditions excluding sepsis. Other clinical signs that may be observed by ICU nurses during patient assessment include unexplained tachypnea, peripheral vasodilatation, unexplained shock,

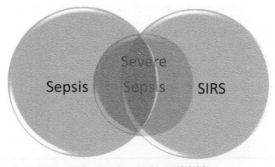

Fig. 1. Relationship between sepsis, severe sepsis, and SIRS.

unexplained mental status changes, and increased cardiac output, with a low systemic vascular resistance.[3]

ICU nurses may even be faced with a patient who displays obvious septic features but does not manifest all of the typical characteristics of the disease process. The bacterial, viral, or fungal cause is often not apparent on admission to the ICU, and positive blood cultures may be the result of contamination. Data indicate that up to 35% of patients with sepsis have an unidentified microbiological agent; therefore, diagnosis and treatment have to be based on other measures and parameters.[1,2,10]

Traditional Laboratory Findings

An increased white blood cell count may be suggestive of an infection, but cannot be used in isolation to appropriately place patients into at-risk or high-risk categories. Acute trauma, burns, seizures, and some medications also can have a significant effect on the white blood cell count. Abnormalities of the complete blood count, clotting factors, and acute phase reactants may also indicate sepsis.[11] As stated previously, these measures are indistinct and subjective regarding a specific disease process.

BIOMARKERS

A biomarker is a measurable indicator of the severity or presence of some disease state. More generally, a biomarker is anything that can be used as an indicator of a particular disease state or some other physiologic state of an organism. A joint venture on chemical safety, the International Program on Chemical Safety, led by the World Health Organization and in coordination with the United Nations and the International Labor Organization, has defined a biomarker as "any substance, structure, or process that can be measured in the body or its products and influence or predict the incidence of outcome or disease."[12] Examples of biomarkers range from pulse and blood pressure through basic chemistries to more complex laboratory tests of blood and other tissues. A sepsis biomarker should have a time advantage so the detection of a systemic inflammatory response to an infection would be diagnosed before clinical signs and organ damage become apparent.[13]

Biomarkers could facilitate earlier supportive treatment and therefore lower sepsis mortalities. It would also be helpful to have biomarkers that allow the monitoring of the immune status, thereby identifying patients who might benefit from a certain immunomodulatory intervention and ruling out those who would not. The concept of personalized medicine (eg, through companion diagnostics) has already been successfully applied in other fields. A biomarker that can rapidly detect increased levels of a specific target of an adjunctive treatment or reduced levels of a critical factor for replacement therapy is a prerequisite for drug development and the evaluation of novel and specific sepsis therapies.[13]

Many of the new and emerging biomarkers for sepsis are components of the inflammatory response system. Most of the physiologic alterations displayed in patients with sepsis are caused by the body's response to the infection rather than the infectious agent, whether it is bacterial, viral, or fungal.[5]

PROCALCITONIN

Procalcitonin (PCT) is the prohormone of calcitonin and is below the limit of serum detection in healthy individuals.[13] However, during infection and inflammation, its levels increase considerably and are correlated with the severity of the infection. In the presence of infection or systemic inflammation, PCT is secreted in large quantities by many tissues. Calcitonin levels do not change.[14]

PCT has become useful as a biomarker to assist in the diagnosis of sepsis, risk stratification, and monitoring of septic shock. PCT has also played a significant role in the differential diagnosis of bacterial versus viral meningitis, and the differential diagnosis of community-acquired bacterial versus viral pneumonia, bacteremia, and septicemia in adults and children. PCT becomes detectable within 2 to 4 hours after a triggering event and peaks by 12 to 24 hours. PCT secretion parallels closely the severity of the inflammatory insult, with higher levels associated with more severe disease and declining levels with resolution of illness. In the absence of an ongoing stimulus, PCT is eliminated with a half-life of 24 to 35 hours, making it suitable for serial monitoring. In sepsis, systemic infection, and severe inflammation, the serum levels of PCT usually increase markedly, attaining values of tens, to hundreds, to thousands-fold compared with normal levels.[15] PCT levels between 0.15 and 2.0 ng/mL do not exclude an infection, because localized infections (without systemic signs) may be associated with such low levels. Levels greater than 2.0 ng/mL are highly suggestive of systemic bacterial infection/sepsis or severe localized bacterial infection, such as severe pneumonia, meningitis, or peritonitis. In cases of noninfectious increases, PCT levels should begin to decrease after 24 to 48 hours.[16]

Autoimmune diseases, chronic inflammatory processes, viral infections, and mild localized bacterial infections rarely lead to increases of PCT of greater than 0.5 ng/mL. In the appropriate clinical setting, PCT levels more than 2.0 ng/mL, on the first day of admission to the ICU, represent a high risk for progression to severe sepsis and/or septic shock.[16] PCT levels less than 0.5 ng/mL on the first day of ICU admission represent a low risk for progression to severe sepsis and/or septic shock. Reported sensitivity and specificity for the diagnosis of sepsis range from 60% to 100%, depending on underlying and coexisting diseases and the patient populations studied.[16] The higher the PCT level the worse the prognosis. The PCT test is not considered a replacement for the performance of other laboratory tests; it provides additional information that may allow treatment to be initiated sooner. The rapid onset of increased PCT level with the advent of the illness and the long duration of this increase provide a broad clinical window for therapeutic intervention. Furthermore, the ease and rapidity of PCT measurement allow swift documentation of the presence of the illness, and permit the selection and stratification of the cases to be treated.[17]

The Surviving Sepsis Campaign Guidelines Committee (2012) suggested the use of low PCT levels or similar biomarkers to assist clinicians in the discontinuation of empiric antibiotics in patients who seemed to be septic but had no subsequent evidence of infection.[7] Data indicate that PCT, more so than C-reactive protein (CRP) or interleukin (IL)-6, is useful in distinguishing between infection and inflammation. PCT values less than 0.43 ng/mL were shown to moderately support SIRS not related to infection rather than a diagnosis of sepsis. PCT values greater than or equal to 0.43 ng/mL support a clinical diagnosis of sepsis and values greater than or equal to 1.58 ng/mL provide strong support for the clinical diagnosis of severe sepsis.[15]

PCT testing currently costs about $25 to $30 per assay in the United States. Cutoff PCT levels for high/low probability of infection are not standardized, and vary between laboratory and clinical settings. Only PCT assays with high sensitivity should be used to make important clinical decisions. High sensitivity is defined as a true-positive rate measuring the proportion of positives that are correctly identified.[18]

In the reviewed clinical trials:

- Less than 0.25 μg/L has been used as low likelihood of infection.
- PCT level greater than 1 μg/mL has been used as a high likelihood of infection.
- 0.50 μg/L has been used as a point of indeterminate probability.[19]

INTERLEUKIN-6

IL-6 is one of a large group of molecules called cytokines. Cytokines have multiple roles and act especially within the immune system to help direct the body's immune response. They are a part of the inflammatory cascade that involves the coordinated, sequential activation of immune response pathways. It helps regulate immune responses, which makes the IL-6 test potentially useful as a marker of immune system activation. IL-6 is an important proinflammatory cytokine in the early phase of inflammation, which increases in local and blood circulation after stimulus such as infection, surgery, and trauma.[20]

IL-6 is produced by white blood cells (leukocytes) and acts on a variety of cells and tissues. It promotes differentiation of B cells (white blood cells that produce antibodies), promotes cell growth in some cells, and inhibits growth in others. It stimulates the production of acute phase proteins. IL-6 also plays a role in body temperature regulation, bone maintenance, and brain function.[19]

Medical researchers are actively studying IL-6 and other cytokines to better understand the normal functions of these proteins within the immune system and their association with a variety of diseases and conditions.[19] The goal is to determine whether IL-6 is causing or contributing to disease states. This knowledge will show how it may be used to help in the diagnosis, treatment, and monitoring of diseases. It may be used to help guide treatment or even as a target for the treatment of these conditions.

An increased IL-6 level may mean that the person tested has an inflammatory condition. IL-6 level is increased with a variety of conditions and has been associated in some cases with an increased risk of disease development or worsening prognosis.[19] Although IL-6 level has been shown to relate to the severity of sepsis and patient outcome, it is not an established tool for diagnosis and clinical decision making. However, studies have recently shown that IL-6 is a good independent early marker of postoperative sepsis or septic shock after major oncological surgery.[21]

C-REACTIVE PROTEIN

CRP is an acute phase reactant; a protein made by the liver and released into the blood within a few hours after tissue injury, the start of an infection, or other cause of inflammation. Like its cytokine relatives, CRP has been extensively studied and is of historical interest as one the first clinically used and most widely studied inflammatory biomarkers.[22,23] For example, markedly increased levels are observed after trauma or a heart attack, with active or uncontrolled autoimmune disorders, and with serious bacterial infections like sepsis. The level of CRP can increase as much as 1000-fold in response to inflammatory conditions, and its increase in the blood can precede pain, fever, or other clinical indicators. The test measures the amount of CRP in the blood and can be valuable in detecting inflammation caused by acute conditions or in monitoring disease activity in chronic conditions.[23]

The CRP test is not diagnostic, but it provides information to practitioners as to whether inflammation is present. This information can be used in conjunction with other factors such as signs and symptoms, physical examination, and other tests to determine whether someone has an acute inflammatory condition or is experiencing a flare-up of a chronic inflammatory disease. The practitioner may then follow up with further testing and treatment.[23]

The level of CRP in the blood is normally low.[23] A high or increasing amount of CRP in the blood suggests the presence of inflammation but cannot pinpoint its location or the cause. In individuals suspected of having a serious bacterial infection, a high CRP level can be confirmatory (**Table 2**).[23]

Table 2
Commonly used biomarkers to differentiate inflammation and infection with normal values

Biomarker	Normal Values in Healthy Individuals	Inflammation	Infection
PCT	<0.05 μg/L	>10 μg/L	>0.5–2 μg/L
IL-6	Undetectable	Elevated	Elevated
CRP	<1.5 mg/L	Elevated	Elevated

Data from Refs.[15,18,19,21,22,24]

Boxes 1 and **2** list other biomarkers used to differentiate infection versus inflammation.

IMPLICATIONS FOR PRACTICE

Until an ideal biomarker exists to differentiate sepsis from inflammation, bedside clinicians must rely on patient assessments, traditional laboratory findings, and emerging biomarkers. Clinicians should be offered additional educational sessions through interprofessional journal clubs to increase awareness and knowledge of the subject.

The ideal biomarker or laboratory test for differentiating infectious processes from inflammatory processes would have certain attributes. It would include[11]:

1. A good predictive value, both positive and negative
2. A method to stratify patients according to the severity of infection
3. A clearly defined cutoff value for diagnosis
4. A method to modify or continue therapeutic intervention
5. An advance in the use of hospital resources

Practice Guidelines

The Surviving Sepsis Campaign: International Guidelines for Management of Severe Sepsis and Septic Shock, 2012[9] care bundle offers critical care nurses and physicians the most up-to-date evidence and protocols in the diagnosis and management of

Box 1
Prospective biomarkers needing further research to help practitioners to differentiate between infection and inflammation

Biomarkers used to differentiate sepsis and SIRS

- CD 25
- Complement (C3, C4, C5a)
- Endocan
- E-selectin (cellular and soluble)
- Granulocyte colony-stimulating factor
- Monocyte chemoattractant protein-1
- Osteopontin
- Pentraxin 3
- pFN
- TREM-1 (triggering receptor expressed on myeloid cells)

Box 2
Other biomarkers that have been assessed for use in the diagnosis of sepsis

Emerging biomarkers to diagnosis sepsis

- Lactate
- Troponin
- Vascular endothelial growth factor
- Platelet-derived growth factor
- Cortisol
- Proadrenomedullin
- Macrophage migratory inhibitory marker
- Activated protein
- CD 4, CD 8, CD 13, CD 14, CD 64
- Caspase
- Placental growth factor
- Calcitonin gene–related peptide
- High-mobility group 1 protein
- CRP
- PCT
- Brain natriuretic peptide and A-type natriuretic peptide
- IL-1, IL-6, IL-8, IL-10
- Copeptin
- Tumor necrosis factor alpha
- Liposaccharide-binding protein
- Circulating endothelial progenitor cells

---

sepsis. However, this bundle provides little information regarding the use of biomarkers beyond the recommendation to measure lactate level within 3 hours and again at 6 hours if the lactate level was increased (**Box 3**).[1]

As of February 2016, a new diagnostic tool named, quick Sepsis Related Organ Failure Assessment (qSOFA), was introduced by the Sepsis-3 Task Force convened by the Society of Critical Care Medicine and the European Society of Intensive Care Medicine. It consists of 3 simple tests that bedside clinicians can conduct to identify patients at risk for sepsis. The qSOFA assessment directs ICU nurses and physicians to look for these warning signs in patients[25]:

- An alteration in mental status
- A decrease in SBP of less than 100 mmHg
- A respiration rate greater than 22 breaths/min

Evidence gathered by the task force indicates that patients with 2 or more of these conditions are at a significantly greater risk of having a prolonged ICU stay (≥3 days) or to die in the hospital. Therefore, the task force recommends that clinicians should further investigate for organ dysfunction, initiate or escalate therapy as appropriate, and to consider referral to critical care or increase the frequency of monitoring.[25]

Box 3
Surviving Sepsis Campaign bundle

To be completed within 3 hours of admission:

1. Measure lactate level

2. Obtain blood cultures before administration of antibiotics

3. Administer broad-spectrum antibiotics

4. Administer 30 mL/kg crystalloid for hypotension or lactate $\geq$4 mmol/L

To be completed within 6 hours of admission:

5. Apply vasopressors (for hypotension that does not respond to initial fluid resuscitation) to maintain an MAP $\geq$65 mmHg

6. In the event of persistent arterial hypotension despite volume resuscitation (septic shock) or initial lactate level 4 mmol/L (36 mg/dL):
   a. Measure central venous pressure (CVP)[a]
   b. Measure central venous oxygen saturation (Scvo$_2$)[a]

7. Remeasure lactate if initial lactate level was increased[a]

[a] Targets for quantitative resuscitation included in the guidelines are CVP of $\geq$8 mmHg, Scvo$_2$ of $\geq$70%, and normalization of lactate level.
From Dellinger RP, Carlet JM, Masur H, et al. Surviving Sepsis Campaign guidelines for management of severe sepsis and septic shock. Crit Care Med 2004;32(3):858–73; with permission.

IMPLICATIONS FOR FUTURE RESEARCH

Although there is widespread enthusiasm for a future role for the routine use of biomarkers to inform the optimal management of patients with sepsis, the field at present is underdeveloped. This underdevelopment provides the basis for the following implications for future research:

1. Standardization of assays for the measurement of biomarkers of sepsis is needed.
2. Studies of sepsis biomarkers need to be performed using rigorous methodologic approaches to characterize the added diagnostic and prognostic value provided by the marker.
3. Clinical trials must be used as platforms to identify and validate potentially useful biomarkers of sepsis in order to evaluate drug efficacy and to generate knowledge on variability in populations and changes with the evolution of disease.
4. Wider use of validated biomarkers to assist in the decision-making process in managing the transition from early-phase clinical research to definitive trials with clinically important end points.[8]

SUMMARY

Sepsis and severe sepsis are leading causes of death in the United States and the most common cause of death among critically ill patients in noncoronary ICUs. Recent studies also suggest that acute infections worsen preexisting chronic diseases or result in new chronic diseases, hence leading to poor long-term outcomes in acute illness survivors. People of older age, male gender, black race, and with preexisting chronic health conditions are particularly prone to developing severe sepsis, hence prevention strategies should be targeted at these vulnerable populations.[26]

Biomarkers play a critical role in improving the drug development process as well as in the larger biomedical research enterprise. Understanding the relationship between measurable biological processes and clinical outcomes is vital to expanding the arsenal of treatments for all diseases, and for deepening the understanding of normal, healthy physiology.[26]

Diagnosis of infection and sepsis is a subjective clinical judgment based on the presence of the criteria for systemic inflammatory reaction, which are highly sensitive, are not sufficiently specific, and are often misleading in intensively treated patients. Measurable criteria could allow a better insight into the changes in infection state during the progression of a patient's disease and would aid in the appropriate and timely clinical diagnosis of presence/levels of sepsis.[27]

When infection is found not to be present, antimicrobial therapy should be stopped promptly to minimize the likelihood that the patient will become infected with an antimicrobial-resistant pathogen or will develop a drug-related adverse effect.[4]

More than 170 different biomarkers have been assessed for potential use in sepsis, more for prognosis than for diagnosis. No biomarkers have sufficient specificity or sensitivity to be routinely used in clinical practice. Combinations of several biomarkers may be more effective than single biomarkers, but this requires further evaluation.[28]

There are several biomarkers available for the diagnosis, prognosis, and therapeutic response of sepsis and severe sepsis. By diagnosing sepsis early and efficiently, patient care and outcomes will improve by identifying those patients in need of acute care, monitoring therapeutic response, restricting antibiotic usage, and allocating resources most appropriately.[29]

REFERENCES

1. Dellinger RP, Carlet JM, Masur H, et al. Surviving Sepsis Campaign guidelines for management of severe sepsis and septic shock. Crit Care Med 2004;32(3): 858–73.
2. Angus DC, Linde-Zwirble WT, Lidicker J, et al. Epidemiology of severe sepsis in the United States: analysis of incidence, outcome, and associated costs of care. Crit Care Med 2001;29:1303–10.
3. Hall MJ, Williams SN, DeFrances CJ, et al. Inpatient care for septicemia or sepsis: a challenge for patients and hospitals. NCHS Data Brief 2011;62:1–8.
4. HCUP Facts and Figures, 2006: statistics on hospital-based care in the United States. Rockville (MD): 2008. Available at: http://www.hcup-us.ahrq.gov/reports/ factsandfigures/2008/TOC_2008.jsp. Accessed October 19, 2015.
5. Esper AM, Moss M, Lewis CA, et al. The role of infection and comorbidity: factors that influence disparities in sepsis. Crit Care Med 2006;34:2576–82.
6. Bone RC, Balk RA, Cerra FB, et al. American College of Chest Physicians/Society of Critical Care Medicine Consensus Conference: definitions for sepsis and organ failure and guidelines for the use of innovative therapies in sepsis. Crit Care Med 1992;20(6):864–74.
7. Levy MM, Fink MP, Marshall JC, et al. 2001 SCCM/ESICM/ACCP/ATS/SIS international sepsis definitions conference. Crit Care Med 2003;31:1250.
8. Marshall JC, Reinhart K. Biomarkers of sepsis. Crit Care Med 2009;37(7):2290–8.
9. Dellinger RP, Levy MM, Rhodes A, et al. Surviving Sepsis Campaign: international guidelines for management of severe sepsis and septic shock, 2012. Intensive Care Med 2013;39:165–228.
10. Ho BC, Bellomo R, McGain F, et al. The incidence and outcome of septic shock patients in the absence of early goal directed therapy. Crit Care 2006;10(3):R80.
11. LaRosa SP. Sepsis. Cleveland (OH): Cleveland Clinic Center for Continuing Education. Available at: http://www.clevelandclinicmeded.com/medicalpubs/

diseasemanagement/infectious-disease/sepsis/#top. Accessed December 5, 2015.

12. WHO International Programme on Chemical Safety. Biomarkers in risk assessment: validity and validation. 2001. Available at: http://www.inchem.org/documents/ehc/ehc/ehc222.htm.on. Accessed February 16, 2016.

13. Reinhart K, Bauer M, Riedemann NC, et al. New approaches to sepsis: molecular diagnostics and biomarkers. Clin Microbiol Rev 2012;25(4):609–34.

14. Vincent JL, Van Nuffelen M, Lelubre C. Host response biomarkers in sepsis: the role of procalcitonin. Methods in molecular biology, vol. 1237. 2014. p. 213–24.

15. Assicot M, Gendrel D, Carsin H, et al. High serum procalcitonin concentration in patients with sepsis and infection. Lancet 1993;341:515–8.

16. Mayo Clinic Mayo Laboratories. Available at: http://www.mayomedicallaboratories.com/test-catalog/Clinical+and+Interpretive/83169. Accessed October 19, 2015.

17. Becker KL, Snider R, Nylen ES. Procalcitonin in sepsis and systemic inflammation: a harmful biomarker and a therapeutic target. Br J Pharmacol 2010;159(2):253–64.

18. Christ-Crain M, Opal SM. Clinical review: the role of biomarkers in the diagnosis and management of community-acquired pneumonia. Crit Care 2010;14:203.

19. Lab tests online. Available at: https://labtestsonline.org/understanding/analytes/interleukin-6/tab/sample/. Accessed September 15, 2014.

20. Iapichino G, Marzorati S, Umbrello M, et al. Daily monitoring of biomarkers of sepsis in complicated long-term ICU patients: can it support treatment decisions? Minerva Anestesiol 2010;76(10):814–23.

21. Kushner I. Regulation of the acute phase response by cytokines. Perspect Biol Med 1993;36:611–22.

22. Mokart D, Capo C, Blache JL, et al. Early postoperative compensatory anti-inflammatory response syndrome is associated with septic complications after major surgical trauma in patients with cancer. Br J Surg 2002;89:1450–6.

23. Clyne B, Olshaker JS. The C-reactive protein. J Emerg Med 1999;17(6):1019–25.

24. Lab tests online. Available at: https://labtestsonline.org/understanding/analytes/crp/tab/all/. Accessed October 29, 2015.

25. Singer M, Deutschman CS, Seymour C, et al. The third international consensus definitions for sepsis and septic shock (Sepsis-3). JAMA 2016;315(8):801–10.

26. Povoa P, Almeida E, Moreira P, et al. C-reactive protein as an indicator of sepsis. Intensive Care Med 1998;24(10):1052–6.

27. Mayr FB, Yende S, Angus DC. Epidemiology of severe sepsis. Virulence 2014; 5(1):4–11.

28. Pierrakos C, Vincent JL. Sepsis biomarkers: a review. Crit Care 2010;14(1):R15.

29. Blomkalns AL. Lactate – a marker for sepsis and trauma. Acad Emerg Med 2007; 14(11):949–54.

Moving?

Make sure your subscription moves with you!

To notify us of your new address, find your **Clinics Account Number** (located on your mailing label above your name), and contact customer service at:

Email: journalscustomerservice-usa@elsevier.com

800-654-2452 (subscribers in the U.S. & Canada)
314-447-8871 (subscribers outside of the U.S. & Canada)

Fax number: 314-447-8029

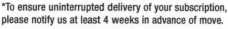

Elsevier Health Sciences Division
Subscription Customer Service
3251 Riverport Lane
Maryland Heights, MO 63043

*To ensure uninterrupted delivery of your subscription, please notify us at least 4 weeks in advance of move.

9780323477376

Printed and bound by CPI Group (UK) Ltd, Croydon, CR0 4YY

03/10/2024

01040390-0010